PROMOTING HEALTH LITERACY TO ENCOURAGE PREVENTION AND WELLNESS

WORKSHOP SUMMARY

Lyla Hernandez and Suzanne Landi, *Rapporteurs*

Roundtable on Health Literacy

Board on Population Health and Public Health Practice

INSTITUTE OF MEDICINE
OF THE NATIONAL ACADEMIES

THE NATIONAL ACADEMIES PRESS
Washington, D.C.
www.nap.edu

THE NATIONAL ACADEMIES PRESS   500 Fifth Street, N.W.   Washington, DC 20001

NOTICE: The project that is the subject of this report was approved by the Governing Board of the National Research Council, whose members are drawn from the councils of the National Academy of Sciences, the National Academy of Engineering, and the Institute of Medicine.

This study was supported by contracts between the National Academy of Sciences and the Agency for Healthcare Research and Quality, the American College of Physicians Foundation, GlaxoSmithKline, Johnson & Johnson, Kaiser Permanente, Merck & Co., and the Missouri Foundation for Health (09-0290-HL-09). Any opinions, findings, conclusions, or recommendations expressed in this publication are those of the author(s) and do not necessarily reflect the view of the organizations or agencies that provided support for this project.

International Standard Book Number-13:   978-0-309-21577-0
International Standard Book Number-10:   0-309-21577-3

Additional copies of this report are available from the National Academies Press, 500 Fifth Street, N.W., Lockbox 285, Washington, DC 20055; (800) 624-6242 or (202) 334-3313 (in the Washington metropolitan area); Internet, http://www.nap.edu.

For more information about the Institute of Medicine, visit the IOM home page at: **www.iom.edu.**

Printed in the United States of America

The serpent has been a symbol of long life, healing, and knowledge among almost all cultures and religions since the beginning of recorded history. The serpent adopted as a logotype by the Institute of Medicine is a relief carving from ancient Greece, now held by the Staatliche Museen in Berlin.

Suggested citation: IOM (Institute of Medicine). 2011. *Promoting Health Literacy to Encourage Prevention and Wellness: Workshop Summary*. Washington, DC: The National Academies Press.

*"Knowing is not enough; we must apply.
Willing is not enough; we must do."*
                                    —Goethe

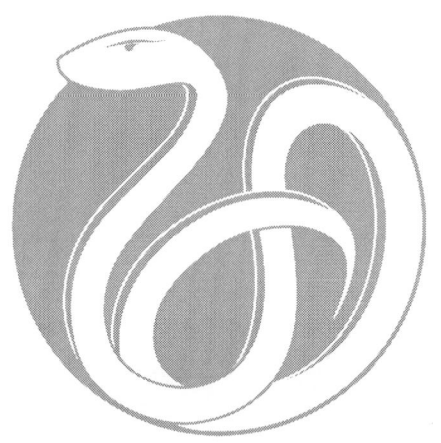

INSTITUTE OF MEDICINE
OF THE NATIONAL ACADEMIES

Advising the Nation. Improving Health.

THE NATIONAL ACADEMIES
Advisers to the Nation on Science, Engineering, and Medicine

The **National Academy of Sciences** is a private, nonprofit, self-perpetuating society of distinguished scholars engaged in scientific and engineering research, dedicated to the furtherance of science and technology and to their use for the general welfare. Upon the authority of the charter granted to it by the Congress in 1863, the Academy has a mandate that requires it to advise the federal government on scientific and technical matters. Dr. Ralph J. Cicerone is president of the National Academy of Sciences.

The **National Academy of Engineering** was established in 1964, under the charter of the National Academy of Sciences, as a parallel organization of outstanding engineers. It is autonomous in its administration and in the selection of its members, sharing with the National Academy of Sciences the responsibility for advising the federal government. The National Academy of Engineering also sponsors engineering programs aimed at meeting national needs, encourages education and research, and recognizes the superior achievements of engineers. Dr. Charles M. Vest is president of the National Academy of Engineering.

The **Institute of Medicine** was established in 1970 by the National Academy of Sciences to secure the services of eminent members of appropriate professions in the examination of policy matters pertaining to the health of the public. The Institute acts under the responsibility given to the National Academy of Sciences by its congressional charter to be an adviser to the federal government and, upon its own initiative, to identify issues of medical care, research, and education. Dr. Harvey V. Fineberg is president of the Institute of Medicine.

The **National Research Council** was organized by the National Academy of Sciences in 1916 to associate the broad community of science and technology with the Academy's purposes of furthering knowledge and advising the federal government. Functioning in accordance with general policies determined by the Academy, the Council has become the principal operating agency of both the National Academy of Sciences and the National Academy of Engineering in providing services to the government, the public, and the scientific and engineering communities. The Council is administered jointly by both Academies and the Institute of Medicine. Dr. Ralph J. Cicerone and Dr. Charles M. Vest are chair and vice chair, respectively, of the National Research Council.

www.national-academies.org

PLANNING COMMITTEE ON PROMOTING HEALTH LITERACY TO ENCOURAGE PREVENTION AND WELLNESS: A WORKSHOP[1]

Cynthia Baur, Ph.D., Director, Health Communication and Marketing, National Center for Health Marketing, Centers for Disease Control and Prevention

Benard Dreyer, M.D., Professor of Pediatrics, New York University School of Medicine, and Chair, American Academy of Pediatrics Health Literacy Program Advisory Committee

Margaret Loveland, M.D., F.R.C.P., F.C.C.P., Global Medical Affairs, Merck & Co., Inc.

Scott Ratzan, M.D., Vice President, Global Health, Johnson & Johnson

---

[1] Institute of Medicine planning committees are solely responsible for organizing the workshop, identifying topics, and choosing speakers. The responsibility for the published workshop summary rests with the workshop rapporteur and the institution.

ROUNDTABLE ON HEALTH LITERACY

GEORGE ISHAM (*Chair*), Medical Director and Chief Health Officer, HealthPartners

SHARON E. BARRETT, Health Literacy Staff Consultant, Association of Clinicians for the Underserved

CINDY BRACH, Senior Health Policy Researcher, Center for Delivery, Organization, and Markets, Agency for Healthcare Research and Quality

CAROLYN COCOTAS, Senior Vice President, Quality and Corporate Compliance, F.E.G.S. Health and Human Services System

MICHAEL L. DAVIS, Senior Vice President, Human Resources, General Mills, Inc.

BENARD P. DREYER, Professor of Pediatrics, New York University School of Medicine, and Chair, American Academy of Pediatrics Health Literacy Program Advisory Committee

DEBBIE FRITZ, Director, Policy and Standards, Health Management Innovations Division, GlaxoSmithKline

MARTHA GRAGG, Vice President of Program, Missouri Foundation for Health

LINDA HARRIS, Team Leader, Health Communication and eHealth Team, Office of Disease Prevention and Health Promotion, U.S. Department of Health and Human Services

BETSY L. HUMPHREYS, Deputy Director, National Library of Medicine, National Institutes of Health

JEAN KRAUSE, Executive Vice President and CEO, American College of Physicians Foundation

MARGARET LOVELAND, Global Medical Affairs, Merck & Co., Inc.

PATRICK McGARRY, Assistant Division Director, Scientific Activities Division, American Academy of Family Physicians

RUTH PARKER, Professor of Medicine, Emory University School of Medicine

YOLANDA PARTIDA, Director, National Program Office, Hablamos Juntos, University of California, San Francisco, Fresno Center for Medical Education & Research

SCOTT C. RATZAN, Vice President, Global Health, Johnson & Johnson

WILL ROSS, Associate Dean for Diversity, Associate Professor of Medicine, Washington University School of Medicine

PAUL M. SCHYVE, Senior Vice President, The Joint Commission

PATRICK WAYTE, Vice President, Marketing and Health Education, American Heart Association

AMY WILSON-STRONKS, Project Director, Division of Standards and Survey Methods, and Principal Investigator, Hospitals, Language, and Culture Study, The Joint Commission

WINSTON F. WONG, Medical Director, Community Benefit, Disparities Improvement and Quality Initiatives, Kaiser Permanente

Study Staff

LYLA M. HERNANDEZ, Staff Director

SUZANNE LANDI, Senior Project Assistant (until November 1, 2010)

ANGELA MARTIN, Senior Project Assistant (beginning November 1, 2010)

ROSE MARIE MARTINEZ, Director, Board on Population Health and Public Health Practice

Reviewers

This report has been reviewed in draft form by individuals chosen for their diverse perspectives and technical expertise, in accordance with procedures approved by the National Research Council's Report Review Committee. The purpose of this independent review is to provide candid and critical comments that will assist the institution in making its published report as sound as possible and to ensure that the report meets institutional standards for objectivity, evidence, and responsiveness to the study charge. The review comments and draft manuscript remain confidential to protect the integrity of the process. We wish to thank the following individuals for their review of this report:

Carolyn Cocotas, F.E.G.S. Health and Human Services System
Norma Kanarek, Johns Hopkins Medical Institute
Michael Villaire, Institute of Healthcare Advancement
Louise Wessel, Association of Clinicians for the Underserved

Although the reviewers listed above have provided many constructive comments and suggestions, they were not asked to endorse the final draft of the report before its release. The review of this report was overseen by **Harold J. Fallon,** University of Alabama at Birmingham. Appointed by the National Research Council the Institute of Medicine, he was responsible for making certain that an independent examination of this report was carried out in accordance with institutional procedures and that all review comments were carefully considered. Responsibility for the final content of this report rests entirely with the authors and the institution.

Acknowledgments

The Roundtable on Health Literacy wishes to thank its sponsors for making it possible to plan and conduct the workshop on integrating health literacy into prevention programs. Sponsors of the workshop were the Agency for Healthcare Research and Quality, American College of Physicians Foundation, GlaxoSmithKline, Johnson & Johnson, Kaiser Permanente, Merck & Co., and the Missouri Foundation for Health.

The Roundtable expresses its appreciation to Scott Ratzan for preparation and presentation of the commissioned paper on integrating health literacy into primary and secondary prevention strategies. Thanks also go to the expert speakers whose presentations provided insightful information and stimulated interesting and thoughtful discussions. These speakers are Jennifer Cabe, Jennifer Dillaha, W. Douglas Evans, Robert Gould, Jeffrey Greene, Juli Hermanson, Charles J. Homer, Patricia Molino, John Montgomery, Linda Neuhauser, Arnold Saperstein, Penelope Slade-Sawyer, and Mariela Yohe.

The Roundtable also wishes to thank the planning committee members for their work in developing an excellent workshop agenda. Members of the planning committee were Cynthia Baur, Benard Dreyer, Margaret Loveland, and Scott Ratzan.

Contents

xiii

FIGURES

1

Introduction

The Institute of Medicine Roundtable on Health Literacy brings together leaders from the federal government, foundations, health plans, associations, and private companies to discuss challenges related to health literacy practice and research and to identify approaches to promoting health literacy in both the public and private sectors. The Roundtable also serves to educate the public, the press, and policy makers regarding issues related to health literacy. The Roundtable sponsors workshops for members and the public to discuss approaches to resolve key challenges.

Health literacy, "the degree to which individuals have the capacity to obtain, process, and understand basic health information and services needed to make appropriate health decisions" (Ratzan and Parker, 2000) has been shown to affect health outcomes (Berkman et al., 2004). The use of preventive services improves health and prevents costly health care expenditures (IOM, 2009). Several studies have found that health literacy makes a difference in the extent to which populations use preventive services. For example, Lillie and colleagues (2007) assessed health literacy levels and their relationship to the knowledge of and attitudes toward the use of information about the risks of breast cancer recurrence. They found that women with lower health literacy recalled less of the information provided.

On September 15, 2009, the Roundtable held a workshop to explore approaches to integrate health literacy into primary and secondary prevention. The role of the workshop planning committee was limited to developing the meeting agenda. This summary was prepared by the rapporteurs as a factual account of the discussion that took place at the workshop. All views presented in the report are those of the individual workshop participants and should not be construed as reflecting any group consensus.

The workshop featured presentations and discussions on selected topics within the broader area of the role of health literacy in prevention as well as a commissioned paper on integrating health literacy into primary and secondary prevention strategies. The workshop was moderated by George Isham. The following pages summarize the workshop presentations and discussions. Chapter 2 describes work by the Office of Disease Prevention and Health Promotion on health literacy and prevention. Chapter 3 contains a presentation on the commissioned paper on integrating health literacy into primary and secondary prevention strategies along with responses by panel members and a general discussion. Chapter 4 presents reactions to and discussion about the commissioned paper. Chapter 5 describes the inclusion of health literacy into public health prevention programs at the national, state and local levels. Chapter 6 reviews how insurance companies factor health literacy into their prevention programs. Chapter 7 discusses industry contributions to providing health literate primary and secondary prevention. Chapter 8 focuses on the potential and challenges of highlighting health literacy and a general discussion that concluded the workshop.

2

The Role of Health Literacy in Primary and Secondary Prevention

RADM Penelope Slade-Sawyer, P.T., M.S.W.
Deputy Assistant Secretary for Health
Office of Disease Prevention and Health Promotion

The Office of Disease Prevention and Health Promotion (ODPHP) within the U.S. Department of Health and Human Services (HHS) is the office responsible for coordinating key public health initiatives, including the Dietary Guidelines for Americans, the 2008 Physical Activity Guidelines for Americans and Healthy People 2010, which is the nation's set of 10-year health goals. Rear Admiral (RADM) Penny Slade-Sawyer has worked to promote the inclusion of health literacy in Healthy People 2020, as well as within other prevention work within the ODPHP, and across other HHS agencies. While many resources are devoted to create information and recommendations, advantage is not always taken of opportunities to improve health literacy by advancing prevention efforts.

One example of such an opportunity, Slade-Sawyer said, is the provision of easy-to-understand actionable health information that addresses people's health concerns and also takes into account the fact that many health consumers must focus attention on other areas such as jobs and families. The focus of public health professionals needs to shift from telling the public what they ought to do, Slade-Sawyer said, to emphasizing the tangible benefits of prevention now and in the future. The Health Literacy Work Group at HHS has worked to develop a National Action Plan to Improve Health Literacy[1] which will provide a blueprint for how health professionals can do a better job of communicating with the public about prevention, and explain benefits clearly and in motivational terms.

---

[1] The National Action Plan to Improve Health Literacy was released in April 2010.

As part of its efforts to carry out this mission, ODPHP has developed Healthfinder.gov, a website that provides vetted, easily accessed information to the general public. According to Slade-Sawyer, ODPHP has conducted research for the past four years on how to better address the health information needs of populations with limited health literacy. Healthfinder.gov is one example of ODPHP's attempts to translate research into information that is easy-to-use for vulnerable populations.

Another example is the incorporation of health literacy principles into the 2008 Physical Activity Guidelines, a booklet that describes the types and amounts of physical activity required for health benefits (http://www.health.gov/paguidelines/). Slade-Sawyer pointed out that by examining the public's needs and desires it is possible to identify multiple opportunities for the advancement of health literacy. Surveys have shown that individuals want to obtain their health care and prevention information from their own health care providers, but are not currently given advice they can understand and act on. In order to deliver prevention information that is easy to understand and use, the National Action Plan calls on clinicians and health care providers to make clear communication with patients a fundamental skill and priority.

There are additional overlooked opportunities in the education system to prepare people to be smart consumers of health information and services, Slade-Sawyer said. Currently, about one-third of the American adult population struggles to understand health information because of literacy barriers, while two-thirds struggle with the complexity of the health care system. The National Action Plan calls on the education system to ensure that children graduate with the health literacy skills that will help them lead healthy adult lives.

The National Action Plan also addresses the research opportunities at the intersections of prevention and health literacy by identifying research on factors of health literacy and by evaluating interventions. Health literacy, which involves the ability to seek out and interpret health information, is crucial to primary and secondary prevention efforts. The purposes of providing health information to people include helping them to pay attention to recommendations, teaching them about risk factors, and making it more likely that they will obtain appropriate health screenings and take other preventive measures such as getting a flu shot. It is critical to carry out research on which aspects of prevention people pay attention to and on what factors, including health literacy, affect their attention. Research can also reveal the factors that determine how prevention information and services are organized and used.

Slade-Sawyer concluded her presentation with an invitation to attend the Health Literacy Annual Research Conference which is held annually and which in 2009[2] was cosponsored by the National Institutes of Health and the Agency for Healthcare Research and Quality (AHRQ). She said that the National Action Plan calls for a multi-sector response to improve health literacy, and that everyone will need to work together in a linked and coordinated manner to improve access to accurate and actionable health information and usable health services. By working together, she said, there is potential to improve the health and quality of lives for millions of Americans, she said.

---

[2] The Health Literacy Annual Research Conference was held in 2009 and 2010. At the time of this report, the 2011 conference is scheduled for October.

3

Commissioned Paper on Integrating Health Literacy into Primary and Secondary Prevention Strategies

Scott C. Ratzan, M.D., M.P.A.
Vice President, Global Health
Johnson & Johnson

In this presentation, Ratzan offered a brief overview of the ideas presented in his paper, *Integrating Health Literacy into Primary and Secondary Prevention Strategies* (see Appendix C). Health literacy is evolving, he said, from the well-accepted definition of "the degree to which individuals have the capacity to obtain, process and understand basic health information and services needed to make appropriate health decisions" (Ratzan and Parker, 2000) to a conceptual framework of activities worldwide. The United Nations Ministerial Declaration (United Nations, 2009) stressed that "health literacy is an important factor in ensuring significant health outcomes" and "call(ed) for the development of appropriate action plans to promote health literacy" separate from domestic initiatives.

To understand health literacy's role in prevention, Ratzan revisited Winslow's definition of public health. According to that definition, "Public health is the science and art of preventing disease, prolonging life and promoting physical health and efficacy . . . which will ensure every individual in the community a standard of living adequate for the maintenance of health" (Winslow, 1920). Similarly, the Institute of Medicine describes public health as "fulfilling society's interest in assuring conditions in which people can be healthy" (IOM, 1988). Public health is not defined solely by health care, Ratzan said, but rather is shaped by what people do each day outside that system. He emphasized this point by offering a conceptual framework known as the Field Model (Figure 3-1), which was originally introduced by Evans and Stoddart in "Producing Health, Consuming Health Care" (1994).

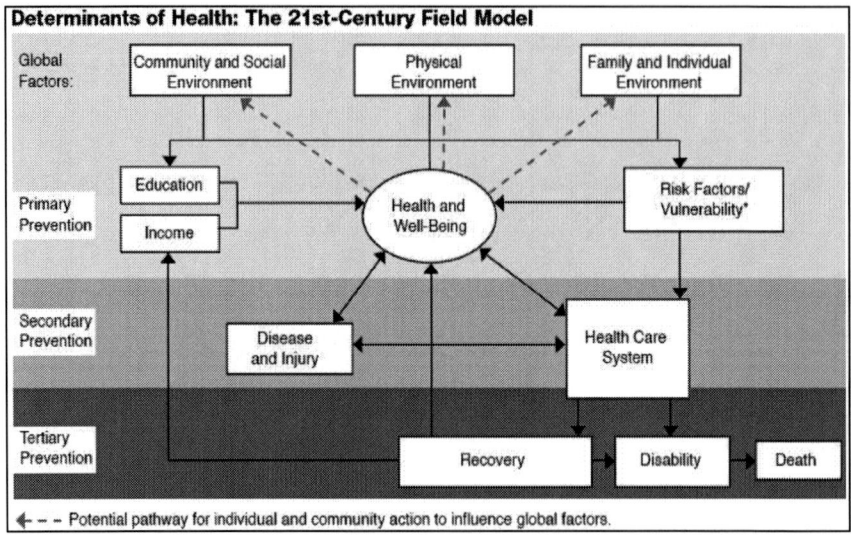

FIGURE 3-1 Determinants of health: The 21st century field model.
SOURCE: Ratzan et al., 2000.

Health and well-being are not primarily determined by the health care system; but the health care system is where most of the costs are. Public health professionals work to keep people out of the system by stressing the importance of primary and secondary prevention. In global health, there is an emphasis on the social and environmental determinants of health. One example is the focus on maternal education, which has led to greater improvements in health and well-being worldwide than anything else, Ratzan said. Cancer, heart disease, and type-2 diabetes are costly to treat, but they can be prevented through relatively inexpensive and cost-effective interventions, including effective communication. Health literacy is at the nexus of creating better communication and education so as to increase the effectiveness of both primary and secondary prevention efforts. Primary prevention refers to actions designed to avoid illness and stay healthy. Secondary prevention refers to interventions aimed at recovery from an illness or injury or managing an ongoing, chronic condition or disability that affects function. People need simple instructions about what they need to do to stay healthy and avoid disease. They need ways to measure or score themselves on how well they are doing, Ratzan said. Furthermore, those who are already living with an illness need information on managing their condition or disability that affects everyday life.

To measure effectiveness of preventive care, Ratzan proposed using a health literacy scorecard which would contain a limited number of key health indicators that are associated with a healthy physical and mental state. Figure 3-2 provides some examples of potential indicators. Individuals would rate their scores against a standard that could have predictive value for age and disease probability. The challenge would be to ensure that the variables selected measure things that are amenable to health literacy interventions.

The goal of the scorecard would be to introduce people to preventive measures and help them understand associated goals. Some scorecards could be self-reported. There could also be scorecards that are state-administered such as those related to lead screenings or immunizations. In order for the scorecard to be effective, Ratzan said, the scorecard needs to be simple and people need to be provided with incentives to improve their health, such as lower premiums for health insurance.

One example of a scorecard currently in use in Minnesota is the D5 scorecard for secondary prevention of diabetes. It evaluates health based on five goals for living well with diabetes: controlling blood pressure, lowering bad cholesterol, maintaining blood sugar, being tobacco-free and taking aspirin daily. The D5 website (www.thed5.org) provides information that shows how well clinics are doing in helping their patients achieve D5.

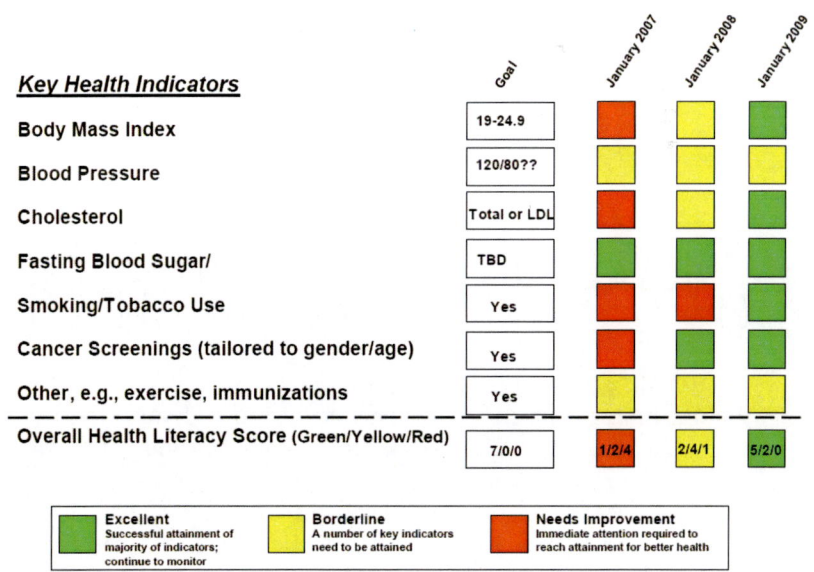

FIGURE 3-2 Health literacy scorecard.
SOURCE: Ratzan, 2009.

Creating a health literate public will be a multi-faceted effort. Ratzan suggested three domains in which efforts can be mounted to improve health literacy: the health system, the educational system, and media and new technology. The health care system can help develop individual and population health literacy by creating health information that is easily understood, by training providers to work with populations of low health literacy, and by making the system more easily navigable. The educational system can contribute to a health literate public by increasing patient skills through all levels of the education system and it can work with people with limited literacy, help equip families and communities with self care strategies, and prepare a health literate workforce.

Finally, media and new technology are useful tools for reaching people with credible and understandable messages. For example, pregnant women could volunteer to receive SMS (Short Message Service) messages reminding them of certain stages in their prenatal care. Cell phone messages may be a way to reach populations without access to the Web.

Ratzan concluded his presentation with several recommendations for improving health literacy. These recommendations are presented below:

- Develop and fund a health literacy scorecard focused on basic prevention, wellness awareness and behaviors, and a system that supports attainment of the prevention activities.
- Health systems must simplify the demands and complexities of those engaged in prevention activities. The Centers for Medicare and Medicaid Services could play a lead role in this simplification. Incentives could be created for health literate communication with seniors. Pediatric health literacy (measures and goals) could be integrated into the State Children's Health Insurance Program materials.
- Define what it is that individuals must do to access necessary health services. Federal agencies responsible for addressing health disparities should support the development of new quality standards that reduce the demands and complexity of the health system.
- The National Institutes of Health should develop, test and implement health communication approaches.
- Health literacy measures are needed at the state and local level. The National Governors' Association, mayors, civic organizations and other organizations should address and adopt health literacy measures of their constituents that integrate primary and secondary prevention into sustainability and other social sector goals. Private-public partnerships could be fostered to create demonstrations and incentives which could be modeled after the World Health organization Healthy Cities Consortium.

- The Department of Health and Human Services should develop, test, and implement culturally appropriate measures of health literacy.
- The Department of Education should develop a health literacy competency base for elementary and secondary education.
- The Department of Labor should adopt a healthy workplace policy that includes health literacy goals.
- Accrediting bodies for health professions should incorporate health literacy into their accreditation processes.
- Comparative effectiveness, including those in development by the Agency for Healthcare Research and Quality, should integrate health literacy into the interventions under consideration, particularly in the areas of behavior change and prevention.

There is a great deal of work to be accomplished, Ratzan said. Two major challenges are to give individuals the basic skills necessary to navigate a complex health system and to work with the health system to make it more navigable. Addressing these challenges will require multiple stakeholders taking multiple actions, including those in the recommendations just mentioned, Ratzan concluded.

4

Panel Reactions

Following Ratzan's presentation, three speakers were invited to provide comments on the commissioned paper which had been made available to them prior to this workshop.

Robert Gould, Ph.D.
President
Partnership for Prevention

Gould said he enjoyed the emphasis in Ratzan's presentation on the cost-effectiveness of prevention. One way to protect the prevention provisions of various legislative actions is to understand that prevention is a way to save costs in the health care system. Gould said he spends his time in primary prevention, and, from a social marketer's perspective, defines health literacy as the effective engagement of the public in getting and staying healthy. He has worked on social marketing projects such as developing campaigns for hypertension, cholesterol, and the Food Guide Pyramid. The prevailing attitude of those preparing the campaigns was that if the public does not understand the message, then it's not the public's problem, but rather it is up to the marketers to clarify.

In a campaign called the Healthy Older People Campaign, Gould said he and his team recognized the importance of crafting a print media campaign that the target audience could understand. Materials were printed in yellow and black with sharp contrasts in order to accommodate elderly populations that cannot see well. The campaign also made sure that the reading level of all materials was appropriate for the audience. According to Gould, social marketers already consider health literacy in their efforts, though they define it as effective public engagement.

Gould's concerns with the paper's focus were in regard to behavior change and using social marketing to improve equity and promote health. Behavior, he said, is not determined solely by knowledge. Therefore, it is important to focus on what other methods, in addition to fostering knowledge, can be used to create the desired behavior. Many people understand the messages and have the knowledge, but do not act on it due to other barriers or beliefs. For example, a small subsample of teens known as high sensation seekers understand the risks of smoking, and still engage in the behavior despite this knowledge—some even enjoy taking the risk. The Truth campaign (http://www.thetruth.com) targeted this population by presenting tobacco corporations as manipulative and terrible, and leaving the decision of smoking up to the consumer.

Gould expressed his support for the policy recommendations made in the paper. Health literacy from Gould's perspective is an umbrella term that means effectively engaging the public. Such engagement is required for prevention efforts to be successful, he said, and primary and clinical prevention are key investments in the public's health.

Charles J. Homer, M.D.
President and Chief Executive Officer
National Initiative for Children's Healthcare Quality

Homer focused his comments on quality, which he defined generally as delivering the right care to the right person at the right time. In *Crossing the Quality Chasm* (IOM, 2001), quality health care is defined as having six characteristics: safe, timely, effective, efficient, equitable, and patient-centered. Patient-centered or family-centered care means that the care meets the needs of patients and families and is communicated in a way that can be understood. This is particularly important in the areas of chronic care and of prevention because in order to make care effective, one must influence behaviors, and the only way to influence behaviors, Homer said, is through patient- and family-centered care.

Quality is related to the construct of health literacy because meeting the needs of patients and families requires clear communication. Clinicians focus on reliable and effective delivery of care, and they are increasingly turning to public health methods of quality measurement and improvement to enhance performance.

The National Initiative for Children's Healthcare Quality places a major focus on childhood obesity and on applying the principles of quality improvement in both clinical and community settings, Homer said.

This focus has lead to an examination of how one communicates with patients about health behaviors for children, behaviors such as healthy eating habits and active lifestyle. Unfortunately, the methods of communication taught in medical school are wrong for effective communication. Doctors are trained to act as the experts and tell patients what to do, whether they are interested or not. Similarly, clinicians have become acutely aware of the limits of clinical prevention in affecting a problem as broad as obesity—what is needed is a focus on change in the context of the community.

Reflecting on the paper, Homer commented that it points out that there are multiple levels of prevention—primary, secondary, and tertiary—some of which takes place in the community context and some in a clinical context. He highlighted the concept of active agency—that is that an individual takes an active step toward a health outcome such as choosing either to exercise or not to exercise, or to wear a seatbelt or not to wear a seatbelt. These actions can take place in either a conducive environment or a hostile environment. For example, the message can be that one should eat a healthy diet, but if the community lacks healthful food options (a hostile environment), it is unlikely that the individual will eat a healthful diet. Prevention efforts need to take into account the context of the individual's environment.

There are also passive strategies to influence prevention, which the paper mentions only in passing. With passive strategies the individual is not involved in making a decision or taking an action toward the preventive measure. For example, policymakers have decided to put fluoride in the water; the individual drinking the water does not decide to take that step. The role of the individual is in influencing that community policy to either support or not support the fluoridation of water. The importance of health literacy in this context is to inform members of the public so that they can influence policy decisions.

How, Homer asked, would enhanced health literacy improve prevention-oriented behaviors in both the clinical context and the community context? In the clinical context, health literacy can help primary prevention efforts by helping people understand risks and benefits, understand the actions they have to take, and potentially, enhance motivation. In secondary and tertiary prevention, health literacy efforts can be aimed at helping people prevent complications or worsening conditions. In secondary and tertiary prevention the kinds of actions required of people are likely to be more complex as are the challenges of communication. Therefore, the need for close attention to health literacy is greater and may require the kind of interactive decision tools in which the information presented is customized to individual risk.

The paper also mentions the need to decrease the complexity of the health care system, Homer said. While this is certainly true, complexity is not the main barrier to primary prevention. In obesity, what is particularly helpful to is to have health navigators understand the complex set of community resources and help individuals access them, rather than helping individuals obtain access to primary care services.

The issue of provider training is also addressed in the commissioned paper and is absolutely essential, Homer said. Medical providers need to be trained in communication in a more rigorous manner than just a course in first-year medical or nursing school. Other health professions should also be trained in health literacy and such education should be required for certification or licensure, Homer stated. Furthermore, health literacy should be incorporated into the public education system to help develop informed health consumers, Homer said.

Additional strategies the paper could have commented on include training consumers and youth in these types of issues, Homer said. Another strategy would be to develop prevention specialists in the community who could work with multiple providers. The importance of longitudinal relationships cannot be overemphasized, Homer said. If one is trying to change behavior, having a trusting relationship built over time is a critical mediator. Another important area is payment reform. Our current fee-for-service health care delivery system is completely at odds with an emphasis on prevention.

Community change is critical in the preventive context, Homer said. One focus of health literacy should be how to enhance prevention-oriented behaviors in the community. This requires communicating to the public about ways to be more effective in influencing public policy, both at the national level and at the community level, where prevention issues include which programs school boards will fund and whether streets will have bike lanes and sidewalks. Successful prevention efforts at the community level are a matter both of understanding and prioritizing risk and of balancing health with other priorities. Most people are not primarily motivated by health; they are primarily motivated by wanting to do the things that are important to them.

Homer commented on the specific strategies in the paper. He would have liked greater elaboration on how to equip families with self-care strategies. In terms of workplace wellness, while programs that encourage healthy behavior in the workplace are important, there are some ethical issues that cause concern, he said. Would employers make decisions about hiring based on health behavior?

Homer also expressed skepticism about the health scorecard concept because it is based on individual responsibility in the absence of community interventions, which can create blame for the individual. It is not clear that scorecards would serve as appropriate individual motivation, and there is potential harm if they were to be used inappropriately in guiding employment practices.

Overall, Homer concluded, it is important to clarify the scope and focus of health literacy interventions, including general capacity, competency with specific preventive actions, and motivation and prioritization. It is also important to decide if the individual interventions will focus primarily on clinical prevention or community prevention even though there is and should be interface between the two. It is also important, Homer said, to address developmental issues of different life stages: parental/ early childhood stage, adult, and elderly.

Mariela Yohe, M.P.H.
Program Director
Directors of Health Promotion and Education

Maxene Spolidor was unable to attend the meeting due to illness. Mariela Yohe delivered her comments.

The Directors of Health Promotion and Education is an organization that represents the directors of health promotion and education at specific state and territorial health departments. The directors administer a wide range of programs, dealing with issues from chronic disease and tobacco prevention to injury prevention, and members have the skills to implement, evaluate and create public health and education programs.

Communication activities have been major components of state health department programs funded by the Centers for Disease Control and Prevention (CDC), many of which specifically address issues of literacy and cultural linguistic appropriateness for interventions, outreach, education and social marketing strategies. For example, in Massachusetts, a recently funded program to improve breast and cervical cancer service delivery through the WISEWOMAN program included a health literacy training component for community health workers, who act as patient navigators or care coordinators for the patients receiving care through federally funded community health centers and safety-net sites. In another effort, staff involved in the delivery of evidence-based health promotion programs for people over 50 were trained in health literacy, ensuring that patients receive care that is linguistically and culturally appropriate with an added emphasis on literacy considerations. Health promotion activities undertaken by the Massachusetts Department of Public Health do not place the burden of understanding complex information on the consumer. Rather, the department accepts responsibility for delivering its services and messaging to all audiences, with an emphasis on literacy and cultural/linguistic appropriateness.

Comments on the Ratzan paper included questions about who, specifically, would be responsible for funding, organizing, delivering, and evaluating consumer education aimed at helping people understand complex health conditions. How would continuity of education be ensured if less-advantaged populations may move frequently and change providers, Yohe asked? The advancement of health literacy cannot rely on the model of the medical home, she said.

Yohe expressed hesitation about the scorecard as a motivator, suggesting that members of a disadvantaged population may have greater barriers to overcome than scoring well on scorecard indicators. She said that perceived barriers to health care need to be lowered but the scorecard may feel like a new, judgmental obstacle for some people. She agreed with Homer that it is important to make sure that health education, which could include health literacy, is available in schools, although it is already difficult to keep current programs funded. Furthermore, telling individual school systems what and how to teach is a daunting task.

Yohe said that she would rather see resources concentrated on keeping health education as a core component of public education for all U.S. children than set up scorecards and other devices that may throw the onus of understanding complex information on the patient rather than on the health provider.

The paper's recommendation "to develop, test, and implement health communication approaches to advance wellness and prevention so that skills and abilities of the population can be aligned with the demands and complexity of the tasks required for health" places an additional burden on programs that are currently underfunded and understaffed, Yohe said. Public health agencies are generally not concerned with educating the public on health literacy, but instead such agencies are providing interventions in the most appropriate health-literate vehicle that they can design and implement. Ratzan mentioned flu as an example in his paper. If one looks at the CDC website on flu (http://www.pandemicflu.gov) one will find programs that address consumers' needs and abilities to understand complex information.

The second recommendation in the paper calls for the Office of the Surgeon General or the Domestic Policy Council to convene and guide agencies to fund and create a Health Literacy P-scorecard in each state. But this requires a set of universally accepted indicators. Which government agency would be charged with developing those indicators? Who would collect, analyze, and disseminate the information?

Concluding her presentation, Yohe said she agreed with several of the recommendations including

- the need for health care systems to develop programs that simplify the demands and complexity of the system (recommendation 5);

- that there should be a health literacy competency base for different levels of education (recommendation 7); and
- that accrediting boards should incorporate primary and secondary prevention health literacy into their requirements.

But, she said, it is not clear how a scorecard would facilitate these recommendations. Also, it is not clear, she said, how quality standards that reduce the demands and complexities of the health system (Recommendation 6) improve health literacy.

DISCUSSION

George Isham, chair of the Roundtable, observed that each of the speakers appeared to struggle a bit with the concept of health literacy, with the definition of health literacy often varying across speakers. This emphasizes the importance of properly communicating this concept to key groups and also emphasizes the challenge of ensuring that health literacy approaches are integrated into primary and secondary prevention strategies.

Benard Dreyer of the Roundtable said he is not sure what to do about the confusion about health literacy. It has been defined and discussed; there are the minimalists and then there are the maximalists. At some level there are people who insist it is just literacy; at other levels people see and include the complexity of the health care system. Somehow, he said, those two messages must be put together in some way. It's not what the provider does but what the patient is taking away from it. Those are two very different things, and that connection is what health literacy is all about at the health system-patient interaction.

In Ratzan's presentation he said that most of prevention takes place outside the health care system. So the question, Dreyer asked, is how does health literacy play out outside of the health system? Food and exercise are a large part of primary prevention, in addition to immunizations. And that raises the issue of agribusiness and advertising. Just as there have been prevention efforts that emphasized how tobacco companies push an unhealthy product for their own gain, perhaps a similar thing needs to be done with unhealthy food and those who produce and market it, Dreyer said.

Ruth Parker, a member of the Roundtable said that the research and intervention efforts of the past decade demonstrate that what people are being asked to do is really difficult for a number of complex reasons that relate to the environment, the culture, and the tasks of everyday living. What, she asked, is the common ground for health literacy that all can agree on? It takes a number of people from different perspectives coming together to make sure nothing is left out, that efforts don't alienate large groups of people, and that there is some understanding of what must be known and done to promote health. Noting that she works in a large public hospital where there are many people with many different needs, Parker said that a simple way of understanding how they are doing would be welcomed.

RADM Slade-Sawyer said that perhaps the focus should not be on communicating the need for good health simply for the sake of health alone, but also because health is the number-one resource needed to live one's life the way one wants to live. Healthy People 2020 has broadened its focus to include the social determinants of health, examining policies in many domains that contribute to health such as transportation, labor, and environmental domains. But the man in the street may not even consciously understand that there are things he needs to know and do to live his life well. Communicating to these individuals who don't know what to do and what they need to know is a very big issue. That, Slade-Sawyer said, is the big challenge facing everyone in the field.

Gould agreed that health literacy requires effective engagement of policy makers across the board—agriculture, labor, transportation, and so on. If policy makers from multiple areas can be engaged effectively and can be made health literate about the priority and impact on health of their decisions, enormous progress can be made. Prevention is a combination of policy, education, and program intervention, he said, even in the case of clinical preventive services. It is also important, he said, to have a HEDIS[1] measure of quality for prevention.

Isham brought up the Health In All Policies[2] approach undertaken by Finland. How might that be applied to what the HHS is considering in its approach to the social determinants of health? Slade-Sawyer said that one of the most important things will be to convince groups working in domains other than health, for example, agriculture, that they do have an impact on health and that it is in their best interests to work with HHS. One of the Healthy People 2020 advisory committee meetings is going to discuss health in all policies and how HHS might move forward with this. Gould said that if the effect of other sectors' policies on health

---

[1] "The Healthcare Effectiveness Data and Information Set (HEDIS) is a tool used by more than 90 percent of America's health plans to measure performance on important dimensions of care and service." http://www.ncqa.org/tabid/59/default.aspx (accessed June 17, 2011).

[2] Health in All Policies "addresses the effects on health across all policies such as agriculture, education, the environment, fiscal policies, housing, and transport. It seeks to improve health and at the same time contribute to the well-being and the wealth of the nations through structures, mechanisms and actions planned and managed mainly by sectors other than health" (Stahl et al., 2006).

could be measured and demonstrated, that would be a useful tool to use in engaging them.

Will Ross asked how behavior can be modified in the setting of prevention-based interventions. There is a repertoire of interventions from tobacco cessation to obesity reduction that rely on behavior modification, he said, and perhaps there is a tacit assumption that behavior modification would also be playing a role in the actions discussed in the workshop, but it was not mentioned explicitly. Gould responded that getting consumers to understand the risk behaviors that one is trying to change may be a part of the intervention. In that case, one would communicate those risks in the most effective and engaging way possible. However, if the perception of risk is not sufficient or effective for change, one must look at other options. Individuals may not be aware of why they are making the choices they make. But if the environment is created so that the healthy choice or behavior is the default condition—that is, the easy choice—then that is behavioral economics at work. The issue may not be one of consumer understanding and processing in order to make a conscious decision. But, Gould said, no matter how one achieves behavior change, primary prevention *is* about behavior and *is* the focus of social marketing campaigns.

Homer said that in the field of pediatrics, practitioners are well aware of the difficulties of prevention and behavior change. One example of this relates to children's car seats. Pediatricians and family physicians thought they were doing a great job talking to families about risks and benefits and why car seats were such a wonderful thing, but what really changed behavior was the passage of legislation that required car seats. This demonstrates that it is crucial, when talking about health literacy and prevention, to include the need for an informed public that can make policy choices that will influence positive behaviors. Such policies range from absolute requirements, as was the case with car seats, to the creation of default situations that lead one to pro-health behaviors.

Gould pointed out that the seat belt law is another example. There is not a person in this room, he said, who would move his or her car in the driveway without putting on the seat belt because it's a habit, a social norm. This demonstrates the interplay between engagement strategies and policy strategies, Gould said.

Michael Davis of the Roundtable commented on the idea of a prevention scorecard. Davis explained that General Mills uses a similar mechanism which it calls a *health number*. The data stay with the doctor and are never used for employment decisions. Once a year, General Mills brings all the salespeople together for a national meeting. They can meet with a nurse for a one-on-one consultation, have blood drawn, and have the 10 factors included in the health number scored. This provides the company

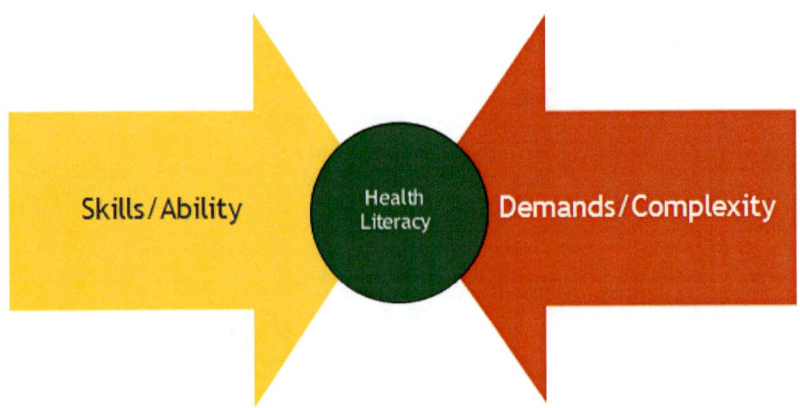

FIGURE 4-1 Health literacy framework.
SOURCE: Parker, 2009.

doctor with an opportunity to create a community health number. Davis noted that if something isn't measured, it cannot be managed. He said he has been able to see improvement in the salesperson community with this technique. Employees appreciate the chance to meet with a professional and are eager to see how they have progressed or regressed with respect to their goals.

Isham commented on the diagram in Figure 4-1[3] which was included in Ratzan's presentation and in the paper's discussion of the social determinants of health. Motivation and social determinants of health are important in understanding how individuals act (the yellow arrow in the figure) as well as how to simplify the demands and complexity of the system (the red arrow in the figure). Therefore context or the social determinants of health seem to be key. It seems important, therefore, to begin to focus more on the social determinants of health when deciding how to measure health, Isham said, and he noted that the IOM report, *State of the USA Health Indicators* (2009) described efforts in this area. Perhaps, he said, one could create a standardized method of measuring health that could be used to engage employers and communities.

Another approach, Isham said, is to look at those health behaviors that are most critical to change. McGinnis and Foege identified these behaviors in 1993 and that study was updated in 2004 by Ali Mokdad.

---

[3] This diagram was first presented by Dr. Ruth Parker at the Institute of Medicine workshop, Measures of Health Literacy, held on February 26, 2009, and it was published in the summary of that workshop.

But a list of effective interventions to change those behaviors is needed, Isham said.

For clinical preventive services, the U.S. Preventive Services Task Force evaluates interventions for their effectiveness. Perhaps, Isham said, a clinical practice guideline that defines the most important interventions in terms of health burden would be useful for health care providers. With developing health information technology, it should be possible to develop decision support systems that take the guidelines into account. The guidelines could also be used to ensure that health professional training focuses on topics and interventions that relate to the behaviors and actual causes of death, Isham said. Then this information could be presented to the public as what should be expected from healthcare providers. The potential to do this is a tremendous opportunity for health literacy.

Isham said that Ratzan's scorecard idea was a good start toward this goal. Homer responded by emphasizing a developmental approach to prevention. The way that messages are constructed and delivered is important in prevention, he said. Communicating messages to individuals at different stages of the life course (e.g., children, adolescents, young adults, and the elderly) require different strategies, perhaps even different messages. Dreyer supported the developmental approach saying that prevention messages and interventions in childhood and adolescence are key to health at later ages. Isham agreed that thinking about prevention across life stages is critical.

Linda Harris, Roundtable member, noted that health literacy is not static. The discussion, she said, seemed to assume that once a message is perfectly formed, with perfect clarity, that the message will be good forever. It is important, she said, to think about health literacy in the age of such information technology as Wikipedia, in which definitions are changed rapidly, not by professionals and experts at the National Institutes of Health (NIH) but by people who in the past were recipients of messages but who have now become the creators of messages. These social interactions, both mediated and unmediated, are changing the landscape of what health literacy needs to consider, she said. Harris suggested that the Roundtable should examine new media and what they imply for a group trying to present authoritative and clear information.

Dreyer said that several people had mentioned that the education system has a role to play in health literacy but, he asked, what is it that the education system should be asked to do? Slade-Sawyer responded that the Healthy People Curriculum Task Force has been working to introduce public health education into the school system. The effort has been under the leadership of Richard Riegelman, who advances the concept of the educated citizen. The goal is to integrate health education into curricula from kindergarten through college.

Clarence Pearson, Roundtable member, said that he is concerned about the enormous task of engaging the 14,000 independent school districts in the United States. Homer noted that districts are currently required to have health plans into which health literacy could be incorporated. Introducing the concepts of health literacy into the plans has the potential to improve them. Early childhood education is another area in which health literacy needs to be integrated.

Becky Smith, executive director of the American Association for Health Education, said that the National Health Education Standards K-12: Achieving Health Literacy was established in 1995. The standards identify health literacy skills and abilities as well as assessments for determining how well students have attained those skills. The challenge is how to engage the education community in the health-literacy effort, especially in these difficult economic times. The past two years have seen a decrease in the amount of health education in the classroom. Decisions to eliminate this education have been based on economic choices, not on health choices about quality of life. What, she asked, can be done to engage local school districts, school administrators, school boards, and the Department of Education in supporting health education?

Linda Crippen, a nurse anesthetist, asked whether the group was aware of how few health care providers know about health literacy. For her master's program, Crippen surveyed health provider coworkers and found that 92 percent of staff had never heard of or been educated about health literacy issues. She emphasized that it will be important to educate providers about health literacy, about communication skills, and about effective ways to teach patients.

Sharon Barrett, Roundtable member, said the assumption is made that people will change behavior because they understand what their health or health conditions are. She reiterated Gould's point that behavior change, not just increased knowledge, needs to be emphasized. Furthermore, it is important to figure out not only how to get individuals to change specific behaviors, but how to get individuals to focus on their health. Alice Horowitz from the University of Maryland School of Public Health said that education in health literacy and good communication should be integrated into the medical school curriculum from year one all the way through residency.

Ratzan said that one thing that concerns him is illustrated by the saying, "The perfect is the enemy of the good." Implementing health literacy into prevention strategies cannot and should not wait until we have perfect knowledge about what works. But what can be done now? What are the options for advancing health literacy? Perhaps Healthy People 2020 is a place to start, he said. Using behavioral economics is an option, as is using social marketing. Isham pointed out that there is real opportunity for integration with the six priorities of the National Quality Forum and the National Priority Partnership. These priorities are patient and family engagement, population health, safety, care coordination, palliative and end-of-life care, and overuse.

Isham concluded the session by extending his thanks to Ratzan and the panelists for a stimulating and important discussion.

5

Intersection of Health Literacy and Public Health Prevention Programs

INCORPORATING HEALTH LITERACY INTO THE HEALTHY PEOPLE FOCUS ON THE SOCIAL DETERMINANTS OF HEALTH

W. Douglas Evans, Ph.D., M.A.
Secretary's Advisory Committee on Health Promotion and
Disease Prevention Objectives for 2020

Health literacy is about health equity, Evans said. Those who lack health literacy do not have the same opportunity to achieve health as those who are health literate and therefore improving health literacy can have a significant impact on health disparities. If one thinks of health literacy as social marketing, then social marketing can improve health equity and other social determinants of health. Health literacy has been a high priority in the Healthy People movement and health communication and social marketing are evolving under Healthy People 2020, which offers opportunities for using social marketing to improve health literacy.

Evans said that social marketing focuses on place, price, product and promotion. When one uses social marketing to improve health, the focus is not only on communication but also on altering the environment to lead to better health outcomes. These strategies align well with the socio-ecological model of health which not only approaches health on an individual level but also considers families, communities, schools and workplaces, as well as media influences and health policies. Childhood obesity prevention efforts, for instance, follow this model by looking at the issue from multiple levels—family, school, and community—with strategies targeted at each of these levels of a child's environment. Health literacy can be promoted for its benefits in the same way that healthy eating or not smoking are promoted for their benefits.

What is needed, Evans said, is to build a social movement around increasing health literacy that would be modeled on other successful movements. To make health literacy omnipresent, he suggested building health literacy as a lifestyle brand, modeling the idea that being health literate is desirable. For example, the social environment surrounding tobacco control has changed drastically in recent history and this required more than warnings about shortened life spans and other health risks of smoking. Social marketing techniques that worked at multiple levels helped change the environment to make it harder to smoke in certain locations, to increase prices, to tax cigarettes, and generally to make it more inconvenient to smoke. Social marketing has also helped build breast cancer awareness and prevention through Race for the Cure, a movement that did not exist 25 years ago.

Healthy People has been making strides in refocusing its efforts to include working not only the public health community, Evans said, but also with the many other groups and individuals who are key to improving the health of the U.S. population. Healthy People 2020 is attempting to build a brand around Healthy People in order to reach previously unaddressed audiences such as the general public, very few of whom know what Healthy People is, and in particular, members of groups suffering from disparities who could benefit the most if Healthy People information were made easily accessible to them and if they were motivated to want to actually use it. Evans presented a framework for obesity prevention (Figure 5-1) as an example of a plan that takes into account the socio-ecological mode.

Evans proposed a scenario for building a movement around health literacy. At the policy level, he said, one could develop advocacy campaigns to promote people becoming health literate—for example, by telling people they can become health literate by doing five simple things in their communities. At the community level access points could be provided for people to enact or engage in those behaviors that are being promoted at the policy level. There could be individual- or family-level activities in which families worked together to become more health literate and to realize the potential benefits for the family.

Healthy People 2020 is focused on building health equity by constructing a multilevel approach to health using communication and marketing both to promote stakeholder buy-in and as an intervention strategy. Social marketing interventions can focus on health literacy as a critical health equity issue for the next decade, thereby being a useful strategy for engaging health literacy stakeholders, Evans concluded.

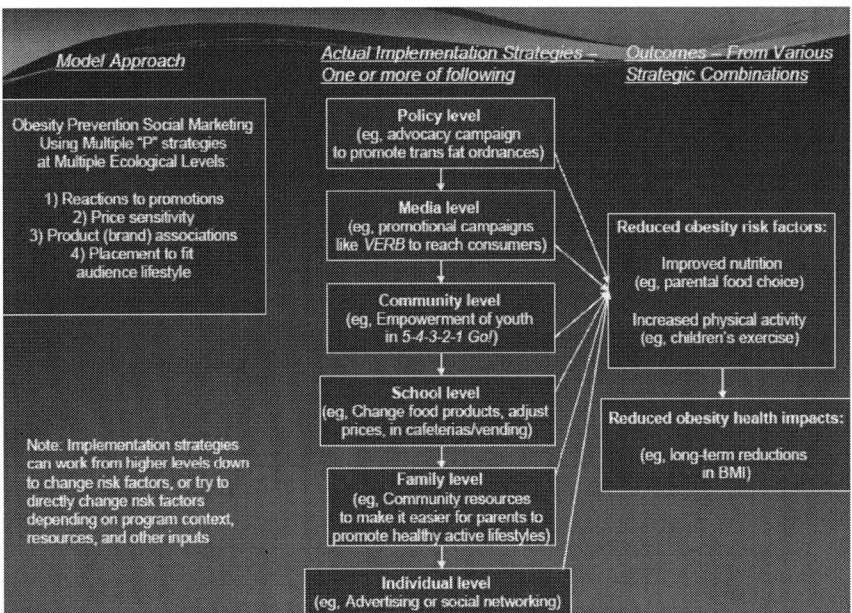

FIGURE 5-1 A framework for obesity prevention.
SOURCE: Evans et al., 2010.

INTEGRATING HEALTH LITERACY INTO STATE PREVENTION, WELLNESS, AND HEALTH CARE PROGRAMS

Linda Neuhauser, Dr.P.H.
Clinical Professor of Community Health and Human Development
University of California at Berkeley School of Public Health

Health literacy is a critical issue, Neuhauser said, and it is clear there are major challenges in improving health literacy. For example, how can health literacy efforts be scaled up so that they have an impact at the population level? What are some of the specific strategies that will lead to success?

As discussed earlier, despite the desired objectives of health literacy promotion, such as those outlined in Healthy People 2020, there is difficulty developing interventions to achieve those objectives. One approach is to advance health literacy through state-level actions. Efforts to improve health literacy could be included in specific laws, regulations and policies, such as those that govern state level health plans or Medicaid. The state level is also a terrific place to educate and develop the champions needed to make health literacy gain traction at a statewide level, Neuhauser said.

Working at the state level also increases access to statewide government budgets, philanthropic organizations that dedicate funds for statewide efforts, health provider and cultural networks, and media.

Neuhauser explained that researchers at the organization, Health Research for Action (HRA), focus on translating research into effective interventions and policy guidance on a variety of topics, one of which is improving health communication. Much of the organization's work relates to large-scale multimedia communication that is relevant to people's literacy, language, disability, and cultural needs. Work occurs at local, state, national, and international levels. The organization has identified seven steps that, when applied assiduously, result in effective communication that is much more relevant to the issue of health literacy and that meets people's needs. These seven steps are as follows:

1. Define audiences and communication goals.
2. Set up an advisory group composed of users and stakeholders.
3. Identify issues from formative research.
4. Draft content using health literacy design principles and user input.
5. Perform usability tests until it works.
6. Simultaneously design implementation plan.
7. Evaluate, revise, and extend to other states.

Defining the audience, the first step, appears simple. But in traditional communication one often doesn't think about the fact that there may be a need to reach and work with a diversity of audiences—not only the patient or consumer, but also providers, politicians, community leaders, and media. One must, Neuhauser said, think about all the different groups that are going to be involved in either facilitating or putting up barriers to efforts to advance health literacy. Therefore, Step 2, setting up an advisory group that includes all these users and stakeholders, is particularly useful. The group members can then become champions of health literacy.

Step 3, doing formative research, is important to ensure that what is developed meets the needs of those for whom it is designed. Using techniques of participatory design, Step 4, to engage the users and stakeholders as collaborators in the development, implementation, and testing of design is key. Finally, conducting usability testing of the information with the potential users and stakeholders until it works (Step 5), simultaneously codesigning an implementation plan (Step 6), and finally evaluating, revising, and extending this to larger geographical areas (Step 7) are crucial to ensuring that one has an effective project and understands how and why it works.

Creation of the California Kit for New Parents, which is a multimedia kit containing DVDs, guide for new parents, and the What to Do When Your Child Gets Sick guide developed by Gloria Mayer of the Institute for Healthcare Advancement (IHA), followed the eight-step process. In developing the kit, the organizers faced the challenge of creating a multimedia, low cost communication tool for the state of California that could reach 500,000 new-parent families effectively and affordably. The kit was distributed at 10,000 different sites including Women, Infants, and Children's (WIC's) program sites. The three-year longitudinal evaluation study found an 87 percent usage rate (95 percent for Spanish-speaking new-parent families) and improved parent knowledge and practices. The kit was revised based on the evaluation and has been used as a model for four other states.

Another example of a program developed using these steps is the California Medicaid Access Guide. California has 600,000 seniors and people with disabilities on Medicaid and research shows that many of them do not know what their health care options are or how to navigate the system. Health Research for Action worked with hundreds of people including seniors, people with disabilities, and those who spoke Spanish, English, and Chinese to develop a guide that would work for all of them. The advisory committee included representatives from the state Medicaid office, health plans, consumers, academics, and professional groups. Usability testing was conducted until actual Medicaid users said that it would be effective. The developers won the IHA Health Literacy Award for the guide.

Neuhauser suggested that the Roundtable could focus efforts on statewide initiatives. It would be great, she said, if statewide strategies were included in the National Action Plan. There is also a need to support emerging statewide partnerships in health literacy. There is much that can be done to improve health literacy by including a focus on statewide efforts, Neuhauser concluded.

HOW HAVE THE CONCEPTS OF HEALTH LITERACY BEEN INCORPORATED INTO LOCAL PREVENTION AND WELLNESS PROGRAMS? WHAT ARE THE SUCCESSES AND CHALLENGES?

Jennifer Dillaha, M.D.
Director of the Center for Health Advancement
Arkansas Department of Health

Health literacy, said Dillaha, is a cross-cutting issue that affects all health care improvement efforts. Health literacy is based on the interaction of a person's skills with health contexts, health care and education systems, and broad social and cultural factors at home, at work, and in the community.

Arkansas struggles with low health literacy; approximately 56 percent of adults in Arkansas are considered functionally or marginally illiterate. Less than 45 percent of households in the state have access to a computer or the Internet, which presents a challenge to information-based interventions. Arkansas also has a shortage of primary-care providers in a medical system that focuses on tertiary care. This means that, for the most part, primary prevention does not occur in the health care setting. Primary prevention takes place in the community instead, and that is where health literacy efforts should focus. Health literacy requires an ecological approach and Figure 5-2 illustrates the points at which interventions can take place.

Over the past two years, the topic of health literacy has been repeatedly introduced by the Arkansas Department of Health and during that time a groundswell of interest has developed. Various groups and individuals were calling for a meeting to focus on coordinating efforts. On July 24, 2009, a meeting hosted by the health department, the Arkansas Literacy Councils, the University of Arkansas Cooperative Extension Service, and the Arkansas Children's Hospital, brought together a broad-based coalition of individuals, agencies, and organizations engaged in

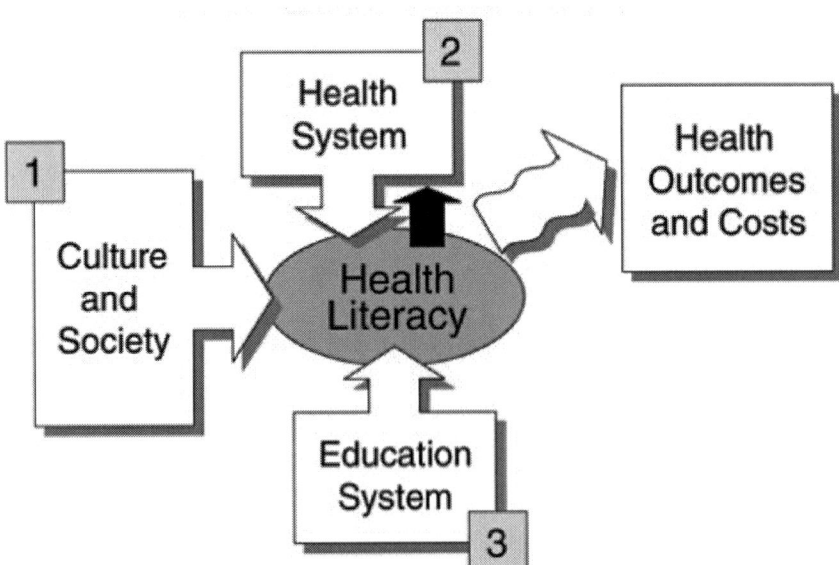

FIGURE 5-2 Potential points for intervention in health literacy.
SOURCE: IOM, 2004.

health literacy—even those that may not have specifically referred to what they were doing as "health literacy." Because of the large amount of interest, the decision was made to put together a summit on health literacy. Planning for this is under way with ongoing discussions of how to partner with others. It is anticipated that this summit will take place by the end of 2010.

The Arkansas Department of Health is centralized. There are no local health departments but each county has at least one local health unit and Arkansas seeks to provide training on health literacy for these points of contact. The administrators of the units work to engage community leaders and stakeholders in talks about health issues for their communities, facilitating a process by which they examine data in order to make decisions about which issues to tackle. Many of these groups are addressing health literacy issues, even if called by another name.

One effort now under way is the Hometown Health Initiative. a state program intended to develop local capacity to build and maintain community coalitions among health systems, the community, and schools; to develop local capacity for health education services; to promote inclusion of disparate populations in community development; to enhance school-based wellness initiatives; and to strengthen local emergency response. The local coalitions develop and implement their own strategies with state support. Key partners in this effort are the Arkansas Literacy Councils which have a presence in most local areas.

The Department of Health has partnered with the Geriatric Centers of Excellence to implement the Stanford Chronic Disease Self-Management Program. The six-week program is essentially a health literacy curriculum, Dillaha said, which trains community members in proper nutrition, physical activity, stress management, how to take one's medicine, how to talk to one's doctor, and how to evaluate new health information. The course is offered at senior centers and area agencies on aging, although it is not restricted to older adults. Dillaha said that the course has been shown to improve health outcomes for those enrolled.

Other efforts include those of the Area Health Education Centers, which are working to implement a model for the patient-centered medical home and are integrating principles of health literacy into the model. Furthermore, Baptist Health developed a new model for delivering chronic care through home health care. Its weekly care conferences emphasize understanding health literacy issues. Patients of this home-based chronic care model have improved disease self-management.

The Arkansas Department of Health has also established a partnership with the state department of education to implement a wellness program called Coordinated School Health. The program was originally funded by the U.S. Centers for Disease Control and Prevention but it has been able to use tobacco settlement dollars to fund one person to act as a change agent in school districts that wish to implement this model. Additionally, there is a comprehensive K-12 health education curriculum, HealthTeacher, the goal of which is to increase the health literacy of all teachers and students. This program is funded by the Arkansas Children's Hospital. The three-year pilot program involves 35 school districts with over 270 schools and incorporates an online curriculum that teachers can review and use fully or partly, at their discretion.

Dillaha said that, because increased funding for health literacy efforts is very unlikely, it is important to work with the people who are in place in order to get them to focus a bit of their time on health literacy issues and thus, to turn them into change agents for improved health literacy. It is one thing to understand what is needed, but it is another to have the capacity to take action. System change and capacity building are needed for a state like Arkansas to promote health and well-being, and reduce health disparities through improved health literacy, Dillaha concluded.

DISCUSSION

Ruth Parker, Roundtable member, noted that Evans' presentation emphasized a Healthy People 2020 focus on equity. But while is it useful to talk about health literacy and branding efforts to improve equity, she said, it is also important to deal with the issues surrounding lack of access to health resources. Many of those who suffer low health literacy also struggle with access. If one tells people to go do something that they can't do because they don't have the access and don't have the ability, Parker said, one is ignoring the realities of the situation. Evans responded that branding and other social marketing efforts are designed to create demand for health literacy. But this must also be done in the context of other efforts that focus on increasing access if the goal is to increase equity because health literacy is an important component of improving equity.

Winston Wong, another Roundtable member, said that the discussion up to that point sounded as if one idea was to aggregate measures of individual health literacy in order to obtain a sense of a community's health literacy. But, he asked, can one measure community-wide health literacy without aggregating individual measures? Neuhauser wondered if there is an existing model for measuring community-wide health literacy, to which Ratzan responded that World Health Organization's Healthy Cities project has a longitudinal grant to explore what constitutes a community, which may be a necessary first step. Isham mentioned Nicole Lurie's efforts using ZIP code level geocoding, but Parker pointed out that the approach still is an aggregate of individuals, not a community score.

With no further suggestions for how to measure community health literacy, Roundtable member Will Ross commented that health literacy is a social construct that requires collaboration across multiple departments to address, since interventions have to be developed based on the ecological model of health. He asked the presenters to suggest how to pull together the necessary government entities. Evans responded that demand needs to be created, and people need to perceive the benefit. Dillaha said the best model for Arkansas has been to use network management. In this approach a person is designated to meet with key leaders personally to discuss health literacy, get them involved, and get them to the table. Neuhauser added that there is an opportunity to create a set of standards for health communication but this will require a champion. Rose Martinez of the Institute of Medicine referred to Figure 4-1 (see previous chapter) that shows individual skills and abilities on one side and demands and complexities of the system on the other side. She asked Evans what social marketing techniques could be used to engage the system side in health literacy efforts. What can be done to convince those in the system that health literacy is important and that there are things that the system can do to make it easier to help meet the needs of patients? Evans responded that the first question is going to be what the cost implications of such efforts will be. One could, for example, develop marketing strategies and frame messages around reduced cost or managing cost—that is, around the message that health literacy is going to be an effective tool to reduce or manage costs. It is known that people who are health literate are better at managing their own health care, Evans said, but that message is not as widely understood as it could be. Social marketing messages could be developed to persuade health insurers and health plans of the net positive benefit of investing in, promoting, and supporting a health literate population and the community infrastructure that would be needed to encourage health literacy.

Roundtable member Benard Dreyer asked Evans how Healthy People 2020 will be useful for health literacy. Evans responded that the information in Healthy People 2020 is being made available online in a digital database in order to position it as a main source of health information. Dillaha noted that nearly half of the people in Arkansas do not have Internet access. Evans responded that the Internet penetration rate in the United States is approaching 80 percent.

Isham said that each presentation was a different way of looking at improving health literacy. Evans talked about social marketing as a process, Neuhauser talked about communication design principles and involving the end user in developing interventions. Dillaha described a comprehensive strategy to engage multiple stakeholders in approaching the problem in a state with particular needs. All of those approaches are needed, Isham said.

What is also needed is a more detailed systems map for thinking about health literacy, because what works in one area may not work in another, as just illustrated by the exchange between Evans and Dillaha. Evans says that the whole country is going to be on Internet, while Dillaha says this will not be true of Arkansas. A way is needed to figure out what kind of approach is best tailored for the community being addressed and that relates to priorities in communities. For example, health literacy is not a priority in the prevention community. Neuhauser agreed that the time is right to develop a more detailed, public health literacy systems approach. There are many models out there that can be used or linked, she said, however much work remains.

Yolanda Partida, Roundtable member, asked Neuhauser if, in the programs she described, there was an effort made to standardize translation of terms that have no counterpart in the language into which they are being translated. Neuhauser responded that adaptation of materials for different cultural and linguistic groups can require extensive work. For example, no word exists in various Chinese linguistic groups for some items relevant to Medicaid. An entirely new glossary had to be developed. A participatory process was used to develop new terms and to explain those in the materials in a very simple way.

Ratzan said, given the different understandings of what health literacy is, would it help to develop a term for health literacy that is simple and easily understood? Dr. Evans replied that it would be ideal to have a clearer notion of what health literacy is, as it is not entirely understood even in the public health world, and that branding health literacy in a simple way will lead people to demand it. Dr. Dillaha commented that in Arkansas there is no need to generate demand or to convince people they need it. The challenge is to provide them with the skills they need.

6

How Do Insurance Companies Factor Health Literacy into Prevention Programs and Information for Enrollees?

Arnold Saperstein, M.D.
President
MetroPlus Health Plan

MetroPlus Health Plan is a wholly owned subsidiary of the New York City Health and Hospitals Corporation (HHC), which is the largest public hospital system in the United States, serving a low-income inner-city population, Saperstein said. It is made up of 11 acute care hospitals, four skilled nursing facilities, six large diagnostic and treatment centers and over 80 other community-based centers. MetroPlus offers almost only government programs such as Medicaid, Family Health Plus for uninsured adults and Child Health Plus. They also have the largest HIV special needs program for Medicaid recipients in the country. There is also a small commercial population which is for employees of HHC and a recently started Medicare program. There are two dual-eligible Medicare programs and, beginning in January 2010 there will also be a full Medicare non-dual-eligible program. The area is small geographically, operating in four of the five counties in New York City but the network has 370,000 members and over 12,000 providers.

Health literacy is important to MetroPlus, Saperstein said. It is extremely complicated for New York City residents to become eligible, get enrolled, and stay enrolled in the plan. Imagine, in such a large system, attempting to navigate through the primary care provider system and obtaining specialty care and inpatient care when necessary. From the health literacy perspective how does one navigate such a complicated system to even get to health care? Health literacy issues also affect members' abilities to share their health information with providers, to engage in self-care and chronic disease management programs, and adopt healthy behaviors.

MetroPlus members are at significant risk for health literacy issues and challenges in their health care. The membership is made up of a diverse population whose members speak multiple languages; at least 30 percent of the population does not speak English and many have a limited education. To address language issues, MetroPlus has about 100 customer service staff who speak 13 different languages and who are available Monday through Saturday, from 8 a.m. to 8 p.m. The automated telephone line is available in five different languages and additional languages are supported through a contracted telephone line service. The Web site is available in only English, Spanish, and Chinese, but work is under way to expand the number of languages.

Sites also have language cards that allow the member to point to the language he or she uses. Member newsletters, which are mailed four times a year to all members, are published in English, Spanish, Chinese, Bengali, and Haitian Creole. There are many other materials used by case managers from marketing information, to basic health information materials that are available in multiple languages. A company is employed to translate the material into different languages, but prior to publication those translations undergo quality review by MetroPlus staff who are fluent in the language. Materials also are reviewed before publication in print and on the Web by a member advisory committee. It is interesting to note that approximately 70 percent of the time the quality review results in changes to the material. The materials are written in simple, plain language at a fourth grade reading level.

Case management programs are offered to persons with chronic disease in the areas of behavioral health, asthma, diabetes, prenatal care, complex transplant, and HIV. Each of these has nursing staff, social work staff, or support staff who speak multiple languages so that there is an opportunity to telephonically case-manage individuals in their own language. There is also a health screening and initial health assessment for all Medicare members conducted in the appropriate language and this has a health literacy component. Finally, there are also some pilot programs, primarily in HIV, that have patient navigators.

In the future, Saperstein said, MetroPlus will continue the programs already established and will also create and identify quality health education materials written at varying literacy levels, in various formats and in multiple languages. There will also be further analysis of the impact of language and literacy barriers on the clinical outcomes of the member population. Finally MetroPlus will direct members to trusted health education Web sites that have the potential of enhancing the health literacy of the membership.

John Montgomery, M.D.
Vice President for Professional Relations
Blue Cross and Blue Shield of Florida

Blue Cross and Blue Shield (BCBS) is the oldest and largest family of health benefit companies in the country, Montgomery said. The 39 independent and locally operated companies provide coverage for over 100 million Americans, one-third the population of the United States. BCBS companies have more than 1.8 million beneficiaries in Medicare Advantage plans and provide prescription drug coverage to more than 1.7 million members. More than 90 percent of hospitals and 80 percent of physicians contract with BCBS companies. The BCBS Federal Employee Program (FEP) has 4.9 million federal government employees, dependents, and retirees.

Florida's population is unique. The state has the nation's largest senior population, the second-largest African-American population, the third largest Hispanic population, the third largest Jewish population, and two of the largest lesbian, gay, bisexual, and transgender populations. Studies show that inadequate health literacy negatively affects the elderly, non-English speaking populations, and also the underserved. Health literacy is an important focus for BCBS of Florida (BCBSF). Individuals who are more literate are more likely to have health screenings, follow medical regimens and seek help in the course of a disease. Children who learn to read by the time they start school are more likely to excel at academics and attain a higher standard of living. Montgomery said that BCBSF is committed to improving literacy skills by focusing its community investments on family and health literacy programs.

Low literacy members are more likely to have more frequent and more expensive hospital visits, to have difficulty accessing care, and are less likely to visit a doctor for preventive services and generally represent a higher annual health care cost.[1] They are also less likely to comply with self-care instructions. The increased cost of low health literacy makes a business case for addressing health literacy and disparities. Increasing awareness of risk and improving prevention leads to a healthier workforce and lower overall medical costs. Integration of health literacy into prevention programs also helps improve member satisfaction. Success-

---

[1] Vernon and colleagues (2007) estimated that the annual cost of low health literacy to the U.S. economy was $106 billion to $238 billion.

ful programs help large groups and employers decrease absenteeism, increase "presenteeism," and have a healthier workforce.

BCBSF's philosophy is to provide engagement and support that lead to quality and satisfaction and, ultimately, to broad access to care that leads to lower costs and lower risks for members. Another aspect of BCBSF's care philosophy and strategy is to integrate clinical programs, processes and people to deliver high performance.

BCBSF is engaged in assessing and improving health literacy. For example, members' health literacy is identified and assessed in care management interactions. Management nurses and care navigators work with members to engage them more effectively and manage their conditions. BCBSF produces all material in multiple languages and multilingual nurses are employed in care units. BCBSF has also created personalized care pathways that lead members to the specific resources they need, and a key component of these pathways is health literacy.

One program that BCBSF has undertaken for large employers is the Care Advocacy and Navigation Program. This involves a dedicated, multidisciplinary team featuring nurse care advocates, financial advocates, and social and community advocates. The team helps individuals make more informed health care decisions by showing them how to use their benefits wisely. Members receive guidance choosing the right care, at the right place, at the right time.

Better You from Blue is one of the company's prevention and wellness programs. In this program, nurses are assigned to members for health promotion and coaching. High-risk members are identified for immediate medical attention and are referred to care programs. The program also incorporates follow-up assessments; various activities such as health fairs and marketing materials. The program is adapted for populations that respond to information in different ways and takes into consideration their levels of health literacy.

Another example is the Next Steps program, which is a regional lifestyle management process that focuses on specialized education for members who are identified early, for example in a pre-disease phase. Healthy lifestyles and behavioral change is promoted. Members receive direct assessments and goals are identified. Members are also given schedules to follow and high-risk individuals are referred to appropriate care resources. Health Dialogue is another program of BCBSF. This program is designed to help members communicate more effectively with healthcare providers. Health coaches are available 24 hours a day, 7 days a week. Educational materials are in various formats and there are 470 prerecorded messages on various healthcare topics than can be accessed by telephone 24 hours a day. In another effort BCBSF has partnered with the Florida Department of Health to administer the Hispanic Obesity

Prevention and Education (HOPE) program. The aims of this statewide program are to increase physical activity and good nutrition, and to promote healthy lifestyles for Hispanics in Florida in order to reduce the chronic diseases and disabilities linked to obesity. The key components of the program include a bilingual website; a statewide awareness and media campaign; free personal nutrition, fitness, and health evaluations and programs; free bilingual interactive exercise DVDs; and access to bilingual lifestyle counselors.

BCBSF has found that health coaching is extremely effective and that patient involvement is critical for behavior change. Effective communication builds trust between providers and members so that patients feel more comfortable and empowered to ask questions and to take charge of their health. Providers are instructed to speak clearly and slowly with patients, to show respect, to use short sentences and pause every 60 seconds, to use common words and avoid medical jargon, to encourage a patient to take a health partner to every health encounter, and to encourage the patient to ask three questions at every encounter. Decision support tools also help members make informed decisions and allow them to access health care advisors and coaching easily.

BCBSF also strives to create a wellness culture. One method is assigning different health awareness issues to a month. For example, September focuses on cholesterol education, and BCBSF creates special education opportunities on this topic for the month.

Blue Cross and Blue Shield is also making efforts in other states to improve health literacy. Wellmark BCBS of South Dakota has created a telemedicine series to deliver information on diabetes management and depression treatment for underserved patients in rural communities and also helps connect residents in rural area with specialists across the state. Blue Cross and Blue Shield Minnesota includes health literacy as a key component for reducing health disparities. Efforts also focus on increasing awareness of the prevalence and impact of low health literacy and on creating a culture where health literacy best practices become the way to operate. There is an annual health literacy awareness campaign, and there are health literacy ambassadors trained in health literacy best practices. Minnesota Health Literacy Partnership involves health plans, medical groups, care systems, literacy groups and community partners to improve health literacy in the state.

Blue Cross and Blue Shield New Jersey funds a multiyear program partnered with the Boys and Girls Club to establish teen mentors who read health-related books with young children in order to instill healthy habits early on. An evaluation of that project found that 62 percent of participating children increased their standardized reading test scores and 65 percent demonstrated greater knowledge about healthy lifestyle choices and nutrition. Highmark, which is Pennsylvania's largest insurer, is actively working to improve provider and member communication, including establishing a language line with an available interpreter and a Spanish-language formulary. Highmark also participated in America's Health Insurance Plans (AHIP) Health Literacy Task Force Pilot in June 2009, which assessed printed member information, web navigation, member services, forms, call lines and disease management efforts.

Montgomery suggested that there should be a strategic focus on incorporating health literacy into policies aimed at improving literacy rates. There should also be research and measurement of the effectiveness of efforts to address health literacy, he said. Health literacy efforts can be integrated into efforts to address health care disparities and also education of health professional.

DISCUSSION

Roundtable member Ruth Parker asked the presenters whether they could envision a competition among health insurance companies to become branded as the most health-literate company. Montgomery replied that if health plans really want to compete to see who would be best at branding health literacy, one would see their foundation arms putting a significant amount of money into addressing this issue. There is a climate of distrust of insurance companies, and working toward improving health literacy may help fix that.

Saperstein said that MetroPlus would welcome the opportunity to brand itself as the top quality company in terms of health literacy. A major difficulty, however, is how to measure whether a plan has been successful. One can measure that an individual's asthma is better by showing that the individual does not end up in the emergency room as often, presumably because he or she has been taught about asthma triggers and how to avoid going to the emergency room. But is there a way to really measure how successful an organization has been at improving the health literacy of its population of members? Isham said that the question relates to some of the issues that Dillaha raised earlier in terms of tailoring health literacy approaches for Arkansas. A previous Roundtable workshop addressed issues related to measures of health literacy and also raised similar kinds of questions. This clearly underscores the need for a mechanism for further work in this area, Isham said. Amy Wilson-Stronks, Roundtable member, commended the presenters for addressing the issue of language and cultural competency. She asked how the plans determine bilingual proficiency for their language access services, and how they ensure that providers are aware of these services and actually use them. Saperstein replied that MetroPlus participated in a program with HHC in which translators and staff were trained and their proficiency tested in verbal and written communication in the most common languages, such as English, Spanish, and Chinese. Unfortunately only these three languages are included in the course so the proficiency of translators in other languages has not been tested. In terms of providers, HHC offices all have dual-line phones that provide easy access to a trained translator. MetroPlus also collects language information on all providers in an attempt to match members with providers who speak the same language.

Montgomery said that there are 100 different languages spoken in Miami, which presents a special challenge. Quality interactions, a continuing medical education-based provider assessment, is useful in identifying gaps in cultural competency.

Roundtable member Will Ross asked what quality assurance measures the presenters are using to identify high-performing providers in terms of cultural competency and health literacy, and what kind of incentives are used to reward such providers. Montgomery said that BCBSF has a pay-for-performance program that uses efficiency and quality measures, one of which is whether a physician has taken cultural competency training. Saperstein said that MetroPlus does not specifically measure or reward language communication ability but it does look at preventive health and outcomes. One of the specific measures is of emergency department and inpatient visits and of the outcomes for each provider. Another, for patients with diabetes, relies on hemoglobin A1C results as well as on eye testing and on nephropathy testing. The measures are outcome-of-care measures rather than specific literacy measure.

Isham said that the field of health literacy measures is not as advanced as it should be. His own organization has performance measures related to language preference, race, and ethnicity but no measures to stratify by literacy.

Roundtable member Benard Dreyer asked whether health literacy training programs for providers exist, beyond those that focus on language, and if not, whether they should. Saperstein said that it is difficult to introduce new materials to HHC and have providers buy into them, but HHC has provided community providers with tool kits on how to help educate patients in a variety of areas such as smoking cessation, well-child care, preventive care, immunizations, and asthma care. Montgomery said that he thinks the best route for education on health literacy is through programs aimed at reducing health care disparities. Furthermore, he said, comprehensive health literacy education should be incorporated at every educational level—community colleges, universities, and graduate training.

Yolanda Partida, another Roundtable member, commented that the issue of language services is fairly complex. One of the complexities is that while one may think of translating material into Chinese, there are actually several major Chinese languages. Translation only covers traditional Chinese or simplified Chinese. Partida suggested that the Roundtable take a look at these issues and provide direction in the field.

Roundtable member Jean Krause said that there were many great ideas shared about ways to involve and incentivize providers in health literacy efforts. But how, she asked are patients involved and incentivized to become engaged in their own health care? How can these efforts become more patient-centered? Saperstein said that MetroPlus does have the Membership Advisory Committee that he mentioned. There are also incentives for members to achieve health goals. For example, if a mother comes in for all her prenatal care visits, for all the delivery and postpartum visits and for the first baby visit, she receives a diaper bag. The HIV program started out giving out telephone calling cards to patients who showed up to visits. Saperstein noted that member incentives are restricted by the New York Department of Health to below a specific dollar value. He also noted that a challenge to incentives is the distribution of the incentive. One must obtain the patient's address and ship it to the individual. With low-income individuals they might never receive the package because it might get stolen out of their mailbox. Even with the small programs that MetroPlus has, there have been a number of challenges to being able to fully implement the member incentives.

Montgomery said that BCBSF uses health risk assessments to involve members. Many of BCBSF's accounts such as school boards and electric companies are incentivizing their members in other ways. Krause asked whether BCBSF will match the $50 million it invested for providers with equal funds for patients to make behavior changes. Montgomery said BCBSF hopes to invest increased funding in patient incentives but, with the economic downturn, it is unlikely the amount will be $50 million.

Roundtable member Winston Wong asked the presenters how they avoid message fatigue in the delivery of health literacy messages. Is there an annual message or some sort of periodic message that is given to providers specifically on health literacy, or do the companies try to incorporate health literacy into other areas emphasized as important to provider performance? Montgomery said he agreed that message fatigue is a problem. The physicians have limited time, they are dealing with all the administrative burdens that the plan puts on them, and now BCBSF is telling them that they need to be trained in cultural competency and health literacy. Physicians are tired of being told they need training for different things. BCBSF attempts to incorporate health literacy into day-to-day interactions across the board. And there are a lot of people in addition to the health care provider who need health literacy training. But there is not an ongoing message specific to health literacy.

Saperstein acknowledged that MetroPlus also experiences message fatigue. While there are no health literacy-specific communications there are quarterly newsletters. There are also blast emails that go out with surveys and other types of information. The newsletter is sent out to HHC providers through the Intranet. HHC is able to measure who opens it and who does not open it. The first few newsletters had a very high readership, but then readership dropped to about 30 to 40 percent. The others never even open it. The good thing is that readership hasn't declined more over the past year or two.

In the third communication method, members of the network relations staff visit the offices of provider to provide toolkits and other information. If providers are willing to actually meet with the network staff, specific messages are conveyed to the providers.

7

Industry Contributions to Providing Health Literate Primary and Secondary Prevention

Conrad Person
Director of Corporate Contributions
Johnson & Johnson

Johnson & Johnson has maintained an 18-year relationship with Head Start, focused primarily on management improvement in collaboration with the Anderson School of Management at the University of California, Los Angeles. In 1999 the decision was made to expand the focus to look at children. Head Start directors were surveyed and asked to identify issues that impede access to quality health care for children. Directors identified parents as the major issue, not because of lack of concern on their part, but because of the difficulties that parents face in navigating the healthcare system. Many Head Start parents are immigrants or migrants. They often face language barriers and are more likely to use emergency services as opposed to preventive services. They are also likely to have low health literacy.

Head Start is a family-oriented federal program that is uniquely trusted by the parents it serves. It was created as part of President Lyndon B. Johnson's War on Poverty and, since 1965, has served over 25 million low-income families and children aged up to five years of age. Currently, Head Start serves 1 million children and families with a $7 billion operating budget.

In 2001 Johnson & Johnson and the Anderson School of Management created the Health Care Institute (HCI) which in partnership with

47

the Institute for Healthcare Advancement sought to provide Head Start parents with the skills and knowledge to

- enable them to become better caregivers by improving health care knowledge and skills,
- empower them in decision making,
- enhance their self esteem and confidence, and
- contribute to reducing escalating health care costs.

The program provides training and information for implementing health care literacy programs.

During the research phase, the institute conducted a survey of Head Start families. The survey revealed that only 20 percent of families had any health care reference material at home. Less than 5 percent said that they would first refer to a book for information if a child was sick. Almost 70 percent of families said that they would first go to their doctor if a child was sick; 4.5 percent said they would visit the emergency room. Once training was provided, there was a tenfold increase (from 4.7 percent to 47.55 percent) in the families who first referred to a book for information when a child was ill.

Since the program began, HCI has engaged in training with 55 Head Start programs in 38 states, resulting in 14,000 families of ten different ethnicities receiving training in seven languages. Training sessions took place in the evening after work for three hours. In the training sessions, parents learned when it is necessary to keep a child home due to illness and how to use their interactions with doctors effectively. An important observation made was that training cannot consist simply of giving a book to the parents. It takes personal interaction with a person who can notice if a parent cannot read, who can help the parent use a book effectively, and who can help personalize the book and make it the parent's own. It takes someone whom the parents trust, who can sit down next to a parent and help him or her go through the materials. That, Person said, is what is special about Head Start and certain other community-based organizations.

Following the training there was a 42 percent drop in the number of doctor visits and a 58 percent drop in the number of emergency room visits. The institute was able to convince parents that doctors are resources, not only for medical care, but also for information and consultation. There was also a 29 percent drop in the average number of school days missed and a 42 percent drop in the average number of work days missed.

While the goal of training was not to save money, by decreasing doctor and emergency room visits, the savings per family trained was $554 per year. Given that there were approximately 9,000 Head Start families trained, this amounted to a net savings of $5 million. The cost of training was only $60 per family.

Following training there was increased parental awareness of health warning signs, a faster response to early signs of illness, use of the health reference book, a better understanding of common childhood illnesses, and fewer school absences, and the parents felt a good deal more empowered. They talked extensively in focus groups about the fact that they had anxiety about their children's health and that they felt less anxious once they had the knowledge the training provided.

Since the initial training, the federal government has awarded a $1.2 million grant for the program to be implemented in Missouri. The way the program is structured, Person said, allows any organization to work with the Head Start programs within its own area.

Juli Hermanson, M.P.H., R.D.
Senior Nutrition Scientist
Bell Institute of Health and Nutrition
General Mills

General Mills is the world's sixth largest food company. Its products are marketed in more than 100 countries and the company employs 30,000 people worldwide. General Mills' mission is to nourish lives through its products. Nutrition means nothing unless it's consumed, so making products that are convenient and fit into a busy lifestyle is important. General Mills is constantly working for product improvement in terms of nutrition profile, and in 2005, the Big G Cereal Division announced that all of its cereals would be made with whole grains. Since then, each serving of a Big G Cereal has had at least 8 grams of whole grain.

The Bell Institute of Health and Nutrition was created 10 years ago to serve as the source of nutrition expertise for General Mills products. Nutrition scientists, registered dietitians and food scientists work together to improve the nutrition profile of products. The Institute is involved in both nutrition research and nutrition communication.

Consumer research has shown that, in terms of consumer engagement with health and wellness, the population can be thought of as divided into thirds. A significant portion of the population—approximately 30 percent—is not engaged in health and wellness. They offer a variety of reasons for this, including not feeling that there is enough time in the day and feeling that it will not make a difference to their health no matter what they do. To engage these individuals, Bell Institute develops materials and education programs that span different levels of health literacy, from very simple package icons and communication at roughly a fifth-grade reading level all the way up to very technical white papers, and continuing medical education programs for health professionals.

Effective communication for General Mills starts on the front-of-pack labeling on its products. For example, many of their cereal packages feature Nutrition Highlights, which call out six nutrients in the product on the front of the package. The six nutrients are calories, saturated fats, sodium, sugars, and then two discretionary nutrients which vary depending upon the product. These highlights allow consumers to quickly see key nutritional information. Another example is the Smart Choices program, a voluntary program for manufacturers and food retailers in which a highly visible and universal checkmark is displayed on packaging to indicate that this product meets certain nutrition criteria.

General Mills also supplies the Women, Infants, and Children (WIC) program and other supplemental food programs with thousands of pieces of nutrition education per year. One example is the website eatbetterearly.com. This website is designed to provide basic nutrition tips and easy recipes with simple steps. The site is available in Spanish and English. While some may argue that the Internet is not the most effective choice of media to reach this audience, almost 50 percent of WIC participants do have access to the Internet.

Mente Sano en Cuerpo Sano (Healthy Mind, Healthy Body) is an interactive program that provides health information and "better-for-you" recipes, Hermanson said. This program was started in 2008 by General Mills with support from other sponsors. It is aimed at young Latina mothers and it is active in 14 U.S. communities. Ten classes are taught and the key is use of the *promotores* model of education. The program identifies a well-respected community leader who is given the tools and education to lead the interactive activities. The program has reached more than 100,000 individuals and the plans are to expand the program to other communities.

Another program that focuses on Hispanic outreach is Destination Heart-Healthy Eating. This is an educational resource that health professionals provide to their patients. Existing materials were deemed inadequate for Hispanic patients, so focus groups of Hispanics were convened to find what was useful or not, what made sense, what was meaningful. Then a specialist in nutrition communications who is a registered dietitian, helped devise the new copy and the content. An illustrator who focuses on Hispanic-relevant images developed the illustrations. The content is available at www.bellinstitute.com.

Children are also important consumers of products and health information. For the "Go With the Whole Grain for Kids" program, cartoon characters (Grain Boy and Grain Girl) dressed like heroes on a hunt for whole grains were created. These two heroes take kids on a hunt for whole grain through a slide program that is downloadable from the General Mills website. The materials provided as part of the program include nutrition messages and fitness activities that can be used by health professionals, teachers and nurses.

General Mills also has a foundation that provides Champion Grants for Healthy Kids in collaboration with the American Dietetic Association and the President's Council for Physical Fitness. For each of the past six years, the program has provided 50 grants of $10,000 each to grassroots, nonprofit agencies to develop programs relevant to their populations. Over 2 million children have been served by this program.

These are a few of the many reasons, Hermanson said, that as a registered dietitian and a public health nutritionist, she feels very fortunate to work at a company like General Mills, a place where people are committed to something beyond the bottom line, to the benefit of nourishing lives.

Jeffrey Greene
President and CEO
MedEncentive

MedEncentive is a Web-based incentive system designed to improve health care and health, and to control health care costs. This is accomplished by rewarding consumers and doctors for using evidence-based treatment practices and for advancing patient education and empowerment.

Greene said that patient behavior and provider performance are the main drivers of cost in the health care system. While doctors have a unique relationship with patients that allows them to inspire behavior change and improvement, such existing solutions as wellness and prevention, information technology, and care management lack provider and consumer engagement.

MedEncentive decided to align the interests of the insurer or employer, the physician, and the patient or consumer. An Internet application designed to encourage doctor–patient accountability allows insurers to reward doctors and patients who demonstrate to one another that they adhere to a number of performance standards. The first performance standard chosen was information therapy. According to a study published in *Archives of Internal Medicine*, patients with lower health literacy had significantly higher mortality rates than those who were health literate (Baker et al., 2007). Furthermore, Greene said, those with poor health literacy were more likely to consume greater quantities of health care resources, which can be very costly. Poor doctor-patient communication also interferes with clinical and economic outcomes.

The issues to be addressed were

1. how to create a solution that would help doctors treat health illiteracy and poor doctor-patient communications, and
2. how to create an environment in which patients would be motivated to become health literate, informed, and empowered.

Health illiteracy and poor doctor-patient communication should be diagnosed and treated by physicians, they should be compensated for this work, and patients should be financially rewarded if they could demonstrate health literacy, Green said. A participating physician logs in once a day to enter each patient's diagnosis. When the information is entered, a decision tree pops up that leads the doctor through relevant literature and practice guidelines. The Web site asks if the doctor is following this guideline to treat the patient, to which he or she may respond yes or no. The second question asks "What information therapy would you like to prescribe to your patient?" For each office visit, a participating doctor earns an extra $15.

Physicians do not like to be told how to practice medicine, so the system allows the physician to still receive the $15 even if the physician says he or she is not following the guideline *if* the physician explains why the guideline does not fit a particular patient. This is done by asking the physician to check one of 12 possible reasons for deviating from the guideline. The physician then communicates this information to the patient and allows the patient to acknowledge the fact that the guideline is not being followed in this instance.

Claims data are obtained from the customer's insurance administrator and a determination is made about whether the doctor has prescribed information therapy. Based on the doctor's recommendation or on claims data, an information therapy prescription letter is generated and sent to the patient asking him or her to go to a particular Web site to receive the recommended therapy. The letter suggests alternative Web access options if the patient does not have Internet at home and also provides log-on instructions with the URL. A user ID and password help ensure privacy. The patient is instructed to complete various tasks online and is told how much money he or she will earn by participating. Once the patient logs on, he or she answers questions about his or her health behavior, reads information about his or her specific condition, and is given a health literacy test about the condition. Incorrect answers cause the patient to be asked to reread information. The patient is also asked to rate the physician's performance against recommended care. Timely completion of "information therapy" results in immediate financial reward to patients for compliance.

The system was first introduced in Duncan, Oklahoma. After four years $181,227 had been invested but over $1.6 million was saved, Greene said. Since the original trial in Duncan, the system has expanded. To measure the efficacy of the information therapy delivered through the program, all patients are required to answer the following question, "On a scale of 1 to 5, how helpful has this information been to you in self-managing your health (5 being most helpful)?" The aggregate score of the 13,673 responses was 4.07. In addition, patients are asked to voluntarily comment on the program.

Greene said that MedEncentive is successful because the process is based upon behavioral science. That is, studies show that patients do not want their doctors to think they are medically illiterate and non-compliant. Conversely, doctors do not want patients to think they practice sub-standard care. The appropach taps into the doctor-patient relationship to generate "mutual accountability" which leads to better health and lower costs, Greene said.

As of 2009, MedEncentive and Medical Justice entered into a partnership. Medical Justice is a malpractice carrier that has agreed to offer lower pricing to physicians who participate in the MedEncentive program and to grant physicians who participate in MedEncentive's demonstrations free coverage during a three-year evaluation.

Green said that to solve the health care cost and quality problems requires interventions that include the payer, the physician, and the consumer. Furthermore, using interactive incentives to achieve doctor-patient mutual accountability is the most efficient and effective way to control costs through better health and health care, Greene said. One also needs precision-guided interactive financial incentives to invoke a state of doctor-patient mutual accountability. Finally, one must improve health literacy through the use of information therapy.

DISCUSSION

Winston Wong of the Roundtable asked Person if there had been any partnerships established between the Health Care Institute's Head Start program and state children's health insurance programs. Person said there had not. He also said that Missouri will be making its actual cost data available after the program's completion, and that other corporations have partnered with Head Start programs in several states.

Roundtable member Benard Dreyer asked Hermanson how the efforts of the Bell Institute coincide with General Mill's advertising and marketing efforts. Hermanson responded that, speaking for General Mills and also as a registered dietitian, a variety of foods can fit into a diet, if taken in moderation. The cereals currently being produced by General Mills and other companies are not as high in sugar or as low in nutrients as they were 20 or even 5 years ago. By advertising the nutritional information,

General Mills not only informs consumers but also challenges the industry to make better products for Americans.

Roundtable member Amy Wilson-Stronks asked Greene how MedEncentive is able to reach those who struggle with illiteracy, who speak English as a second language, or who have other barriers to using a Web application. Greene said that during the first year in Duncan, the city put a kiosk at the city hall and there was a steady flow of individuals, many of whom were not computer-literate or did not know how to use computers. That year the participation rate was about 43 percent. MedEncentive urges insurance providers to encourage employees within plans and their beneficiaries who do not speak English or who have difficulties with computers, to reach out to friends and family members who can help. He also said that for the right financial incentive, he believes people will find a way to participate. As time goes on, Greene said, information therapy is being delivered through video and audio messages which, it is hoped, will circumvent some of these literacy issues.

Cynthia Baur of the Centers for Disease Control and Prevention said that because of strict regulations public health agencies find it very difficult to conduct the kinds of consumer research that private companies do. She asked if there was a way to build partnerships between consumer product companies and public health agencies to do research that helps everyone better understand people's needs and wants. Hermanson responded that it is probably true that consumer product companies have extensive data that help the companies craft messages to be relevant for consumers, in order to reach the populations the companies want to target. General Mills would, she said, be open to continuing the dialogue begun at this workshop.

Another participant asked Greene if physician offices need to have electronic medical records in place to participate in MedEncentive. Greene replied that the system is designed to be flexible so that it can be used in either low-tech or high-tech environments. For example, doctors can handwrite their responses for nurses to enter, as long as the nurse is enrolled in the program under the supervision of the physician. On the other end of the spectrum, some doctors have integrated the program with their tablets so that when a beneficiary arrives at the practice, a MedEncentive icon pops up to alert the physician to the presence of a relevant guideline.

Isham said that he was impressed by the ingenuity of the three approaches discussed by this panel. On the one hand, there is the Head Start program that reaches out and educates a vulnerable segment of the population. Then there is the program from MedEncentive which attempts to triangulate incentives for three major stakeholders—the physician, the consumer, and the insurer. Finally, there is a large consumer product corporation that is teaching how to segment, label, and help people to make choices. That kind of combination of talent and approaches are needed, as is good science, Isham said, in order to make progress on health literacy.

8

The Potential and Challenges of Highlighting Health Literacy

Jennifer Cabe, M.A.
Executive Director
Canyon Ranch Institute

The health in all policies focus mentioned by Slade-Sawyer earlier originally led to the interest and involvement of the Office of the Surgeon General in health literacy activities. Dr. Richard Carmona, 17th Surgeon General (2002-2006), identified health literacy as a topic of major importance, making it a topic of prominence for the Office of the Surgeon General. There was a realization that health literacy could have a major impact in the field of health communication and that it could affect health behavior and produce real physical and physiological changes not only in individuals but across a population. The question faced by the Office of the Surgeon General was how to infuse health literacy into every aspect of prevention, preparedness, and the elimination of health disparities.

While the reports from the Office of Surgeon General are wonderful reports that bring together the science on a topic, Dr. Carmona questioned who was reading and using them. This led to the idea of developing what he called the People's Piece, an approach that has continued. Peoples Pieces are issued with full Surgeon General reports and Calls to Action. They are released online and in print, and are written at fifth- or sixth-grade reading levels. They have been translated into numerous languages and distributed by the government, by health insurers, and by states. Major magazines, such as *Good Housekeeping*, have published them in their entirety.

After leaving the position of Surgeon General, Dr. Carmona took the ideas and concepts he had been working with to the Canyon Ranch Institute, a nonprofit organization whose mission is to help educate, inspire and empower every person to prevent disease and embrace wellness. The Canyon Ranch Institute views health literacy as

- a tool for prevention and better care;
- important for clinical, public health, K-12 education, adult literacy, care advocacy and navigation, and workplace wellness and workforce productivity;
- including the skills and abilities that determine the extent that *all people* can find, understand, evaluate, communicate, and use health information; and
- leading to informed choices, reduced health risks, better navigation of the existing health care system, reduced inequities in health, and increased quality of life.

Health literacy is not about communicating health for health's sake, Cabe said, but rather about communicating health in the context of what people need to know. This applies to individuals, parents, educators, health care professionals, health care systems, policy makers and policy brokers, government staff and officials, media, and community leaders.

In the ongoing debate about health care reform there is an opportunity to make prevention as great a priority as treatment, and to recognize the contributions of health literacy to both. Investment in the avoidable causes of mortality, that is in prevention efforts, are dwarfed by our investment in medical care and biomedical research. Health care reform, Cabe said, is an opportunity to focus the system on prevention rather than sick care.

Chronic diseases account for more than 75 cents of every dollar spent on health care in the United States. Yet most chronic diseases are preventable or manageable with appropriate preventive efforts. If one were the chief executive officer of a company and realized that 75 percent of company spending was unnecessary, it would be time to determine how to stop the waste. Prevention can eliminate unnecessary spending as well as save lives and reduce and eliminate suffering from many diseases that are completely preventable, Cabe said. Health literacy can lead the way, she said, and she proposed some strategies:

- Communicate at the appropriate literacy level for the audience.
- Create health literacy courses in Adult Basic Education, in K-12, and in training of all health care workers.
  - o   Establish health literacy learning standards across the lifespan.

- Establish health literacy centers of excellence for each state.
- Incorporate health literacy in all health and medical certification courses.
- Incorporate health literacy into national health surveillance efforts.
  o First, fund development of a comprehensive measure of health literacy.
- Build demonstration projects specifically targeting reductions in health disparities by using health literacy.
  o Specifically target changes in cost, health status, equity, and sustainability issues as priority outcome areas.
- Create and monitor standards for hospital operations (via Joint Commission).
  o Mandate local participation on evaluation teams.
- Emphasize health literacy as a solution in Healthy People 2020 goals.

As mentioned earlier, the study discussed by Crippen found that over 90 percent of health professionals in the study did not know anything about health literacy. Yet there are programs that are going on around the country and around the world to train health professionals in health literacy. Perhaps one of the things that should be done is to examine the outcomes of that training. Cabe also said that it is crucial to get health literacy into health professional certification and licensure tests.

The Canyon Ranch Institute views the advancement of health literacy as crucial to creating a preventive care system. To highlight health literacy in prevention programs means more than just ensuring that programs are accessible to people with low health literacy. It means

- designing programs to advance health literacy;
- prospectively identifying and then measuring outcomes in health literacy, behavior, physical changes, and physiological changes;
- measuring process and program effectiveness and adapting to the needs of all partners and participants;
- preventing disease;
- improving health and well-being; and
- eliminating health disparities.

The Institute organized an integrated health literacy training program, the Life Enhancement Program, at the Urban Health Plan, a community health center in the South Bronx that serves 28,000 patients. One of the things needed was a place to hold the program so within the community health center building a health and wellness center was designed and built. The curriculum, which contained information on nutrition, physical activity, integrative medicine, and social support, was taught first to the center's staff and leadership and then to patients. Staff involved in the training included the chief medical officer, a nutritionist, a social worker, a physical therapist, an exercise physiologist, the person in charge of public health and continuous quality improvement, a psychiatrist, and the center's chief executive officer.

During the training, the health professionals learned how to communicate key messages to their patients. They also learned that healthy messages have to be achievable. For example, if a patient is told to eat more fresh fruits and vegetables but does not have access to such food, it does more harm than good. Since that was one message that was going to be conveyed to patients, the center worked with a local bodega to get it to stock healthy foods in addition to the items such as chips and liquor that were its standard fare.

Most of the people who participated in the program were not engaged in any sort of physical activity at the beginning. But they began to use the equipment in the health and wellness center. They also said they wanted to do something even closer to their hearts, and that is when the Latin dance program at Urban Health Plan was started and included as part of this program.

The Institute measured outcomes of the program, Cabe said. At the community level many participants reported sharing the program guide (a book with information about nutrition, physical activity, and other health information) with their family members and their neighbors. It was in Spanish, and it was something that they liked, so they shared it. Changes in health literacy skills and behavior included improved nutrition habits, increased physical activity, and improved interaction among health care professionals and patients. Patients learned that they could prepare for a visit to the physician, that they could ask questions. Health outcomes included weight loss and stress reduction. Suggestions for improving the program included a desire for more time, more scientific information (e.g., how nutrition affects the body), and the use of more charts and graphs.

At no time during the program did any of the health professionals or any of the patients say that they wanted incentives, such as payment or gifts, in order to participate in the program, Cabe said. The first patient participants in the program were referred by their physicians. But referrals are no longer necessary to fill the program. Patients who have gone through the program are recruiting their family members and their friends to participate.

Canyon Ranch Institute is beginning to look at making the business case for health literacy, Cabe said. It is also important to measure the sustainability of changes achieved. The scorecard idea is worth pursuing if it is used in the context of a community-based, integrative health model such as that of the institute or the Head Start program described earlier, but the scorecard must be uniform and reflect community needs.

To succeed, Cabe said, health literacy efforts will need to engage in partnerships with invested stakeholders. Health literacy should be proactive, not reactive. Health literacy is prevention, Cabe said, and it can save lives and save money.

References

Baker, D. W., M. S. Wolf, J. Feinglass, J. A. Thompson, J.A. Gazmararian, and H. Jenny. 2007. Health Literacy and Mortality Among Elderly Persons. *Archives of Internal Medicine* 167(14):1503-1509.

Berkman, N. D., D. A. Dewalt M. Pignone S. L. Sherida K. N. Lohr L. Lux S. F. Sutton, T. Swinson and A. J. Bonito. 2004. Literacy and health outcomes. *Evidence Report/Technology Assessment* (87):1-8.

Evans, R. G., and G. L. Stoddart. 1994. Producing health, consuming health care. In *Why are some people healthy and others not? The determinants of health of populations*, edited by R. G. Evans, M. L. Barer and T. R. Marmor. New York: Aldine de Gruyter.

Evans, W. D., K. K. Christoffel, J. W. Necheles, and A. B. Becker. 2010. Social marketing as a childhood obesity prevention strategy. *Obesity* 18(n1s):S23-S26.

IOM (Institute of Medicine). 1988. *The future of public health.* Washington, DC: National Academy Press.

IOM. 2001. *Crossing the Quality Chasm.* Washington, DC: National Academy Press.

IOM. 2004. *Health literacy: A prescription to end confusion.* Washington, DC: The National Academies Press.

IOM. 2009. *State of the USA health indicators: Letter report.* Washington, DC: The National Academies Press.

Lillie, S. E., N. T. Brewer, S. C. O'Neill, E. G. Morrill, E. C. Dees, L. A. Carey, and B. K. Rimer. 2007. Retention and use of breast cancer recurrence risk information from genomic tests: the role of health literacy. *Cancer Epidemiology, Biomarkers & Prevention* 16(2): 249-255.

Montgomery, J. M. 2009. IOM roundtable on health literacy: How the Blue Cross Blue Shield system factors health literacy into prevention programs. PowerPoint presentation at the Institute of Medicine workshop on integrating health literacy into prevention programs, Washington, DC. September 15.

Parker, R. 2009. Measuring health literacy: What? So What? Now What? PowerPoint presentation at the Institute of Medicine workshop on measures of health literacy. Washington, DC, February 26.

Ratzan, S. C. 2009. *Integrating Health Literacy into Primary and Secondary Prevention Strategies*. PowerPoint presentation at the Institute of Medicine Workshop on Integrating Health Literacy into Primary and Secondary Prevention Strategies.

Ratzan, S., and R. Parker. 2000. Introduction. In *National Library of Medicine current bibliographies in medicine: Health literacy*. NLM Pub. No. CBM 2000-1 ed, edited by C. Selden, M. Zorn, S. Ratzan and R. Parker. Bethesda, MD: National Institutes of Health, U.S. Department of Health and Human Services.

Ratzan, S. C., G. L. Filerman, and J. W. LeSar. 2000. Attaining global health: Challenges and opportunities. *Population Bulletin* 55(1):1-48.

Stahl, T., M. Wismar, E. Ollila, E. Lahtinen, and K. Leppor. 2006. *Health in All Policies: Prospects and Potentials*. Ministry of Social Affairs and Health. Finland.

United Nations. 2009. *Ministerial declaration*. http://www.un.org/en/ecosoc/julyhls/pdf09/ministerial_declaration-2009.pdf (accessed 2009).

Vernon, J., A. Trujillo, S. Rosenbaum, and B. DeBuouno. 2007. Low Health Literacy: Implications for National Policy. A http://www.npsf.org/askme3/download/UCONN_Health%20Literacy%20Report.pdf.

Winslow, C. 1920. The untilled field of public health. *Modern Medicine* 2:183-191.

Appendix A

Workshop Agenda

Tuesday, September 15, 2009
7:45 am-5:15 pm
Adams & Franklin Room
Washington Plaza Hotel
10 Thomas Circle, NW
Washington, DC

AGENDA

CLOSED SESSION   Diplomat Room (2nd Floor)

7:45-8:30 am   Roundtable Breakfast

OPEN SESSION   WORKSHOP   Adams & Franklin Room (1st Floor)

9:00-9:15 am   Welcome and Overview
                    George J. Isham, M.D., M.S.
                    Chair, Roundtable on Health Literacy
                    Chief Health Officer and Plan Medical Director
                    HealthPartners

9:15-9:30 am   The Role of Health Literacy in Primary and Secondary
                Prevention
                    RADM Penelope Slade-Sawyer, P.T., M.S.W.
                    Deputy Assistant Secretary of Health
                    Disease Prevention and Health Promotion
                    Director, Office of Disease Prevention and Health
                    Promotion
                    Office of Public Health and Science
                    U.S. Department of Health and Human Services

9:30-9:50 am   Commissioned Paper on Integrating Health Literacy
                into Primary and Secondary Prevention Strategies
                (Includes both evidence-based information and theories
                of how effective integration could occur.)
                    Scott C. Ratzan, M.D., M.P.A.
                    Vice President, Global Health
                    Johnson & Johnson

9:50-10:30 am   **Panel Reactions**
                (Each presenter will have 10-15 minutes.)

                Partnership for Prevention
                    Robert Gould, Ph.D.
                    President

                National Initiative for Children's Healthcare Quality
                    Charles J. Homer, M.D.
                    President and CEO

                Directors of Health Promotion and Education
                    Mariela Yohe, M.P.H.
                    Program Director

10:30-11:30 am Discussion

11:30 am-   ROUNDTABLE LUNCH   1st Floor Lounge
12:30 pm

12:30-1:15 pm   **Panel: Intersection of Health Literacy and Public
                Health Prevention Programs**
                (Each presenter will have 15 minutes.)

National: Incorporating Health Literacy into the
Healthy People Focus on the Social Determinants of
Health.
W. Douglas Evans, Ph.D., M.A.
Member
Secretary's Advisory Committee on Health
Promotion and Disease Prevention Objectives for
2020

State: How Have the Concepts of Health Literacy Been
Incorporated into State Prevention, Wellness, and
Health Care Programs? What Are the Successes and
Challenges?
Linda Neuhauser, Dr.P.H.
Clinical Professor of Community Health and Human
Development
School of Public Health
University of California, Berkeley
Co-Principal Investigator
Health Research for Action Center

Local: How Have the Concepts of Health Literacy
Been Incorporated into Local Prevention and Wellness
Programs? What Are the Successes and Challenges?
Jennifer Dillaha, M.D.
Director of the Center for Health Advancement
Arkansas Department of Health

1:15-1:45 pm   Discussion

1:45-2:30 pm   **Panel: How Do Insurance Companies, Especially
Managed Care Insurance Companies, Factor in Health
Literacy in the Creation of Their Prevention Programs
and Their Preventative Information for Their
Enrollees?**
(Each participant will have 15 minutes.)

MetroPlus Health Plan
Arnold Saperstein, M.D.
President

Blue Cross and Blue Shield
John Montgomery, M.D.
Vice President for Professional Relations
Blue Cross and Blue Shield of Florida

2:30-3:00 pm   Discussion

3:00-3:15 pm   BREAK

3:15-4:00 pm   **Panel: Industry Contributions to Providing Health Literate Primary and Secondary Prevention**
(Each participant will have 15 minutes.)

General Mills
Juli Hermanson, M.P.H., R.D.
Senior Nutrition Scientist
Bell Institute of Health and Nutrition

MedEncentive
Jeffrey Greene
President and CEO

4:00-4:30 pm   Discussion

4:30-4:50 pm   The Potential and Challenges of Highlighting Health Literacy
Jennifer Cabe, M.A.
Executive Director
Canyon Ranch Institute

4:50-5:15 pm   Discussion

5:15 pm   ADJOURN WORKSHOP

Appendix B

Workshop Speaker Biosketches

Jennifer Cabe, M.A., is executive director of the Canyon Ranch Institute. Prior to joining Canyon Ranch Institute in 2007, Ms. Cabe was vice president of Scientific Communications for Feinstein Kean Healthcare. She previously served in the Office of the Surgeon General as communications director and speechwriter for Surgeon General Richard H. Carmona. Prior to joining the Office of the Surgeon General, Ms. Cabe was the communications officer at the Fogarty International Center at the National Institutes of Health in Bethesda, Maryland, and had communications, wellness, and government relations for HealthNet Health Plan in the Pacific Northwest. She was also the founder and publisher of *Best of Health & Fitness,* a successful national customized magazine for the health and fitness industry.

Ms. Cabe was awarded the Surgeon General's Medallion in 2005 and has also received the U.S. Department of Health and Human Services Honor Award for her role in developing the "U.S. Surgeon General's Family History Initiative." Since then, she has received numerous awards including the National Institutes of Health Team Merit Award (2006). Ms. Cabe earned a bachelor's degree at Trinity University in San Antonio, Texas, and a master's in public communication with an emphasis in health communication at American University in Washington, DC.

Jennifer Dillaha, M.D., is the director of the Center for Health Advancement for the Arkansas Department of Health. Since joining the Health Department in 2001, she has played a leading role in the Agency's health promotion efforts, using a life stage approach that focuses on population-based interventions to reduce the burden of chronic disease among all Arkansans. Under her leadership, the Health Department has made improving health literacy a cross-cutting strategic priority that is fundamental to its prevention efforts. Dr. Dillaha is a physician with specialty training in internal medicine and subspecialty training in infectious diseases and in geriatric medicine. She also has faculty appointments as an assistant professor in the University of Arkansas for Medical Sciences College of Public Health and College of Medicine.

W. Douglas Evans, Ph.D., M.A., is director of Public Health Communication and Marketing, and professor in the Department of Prevention and Community Health and the Department of Global Health at the George Washington School of Public Health and Health Services. A research psychologist, his work focuses on two key areas: building the evidence base to establish the effectiveness of marketing and message strategies in promoting healthy behaviors and expanding the use of effective commercial marketing strategies to public health, especially to reach socially and economically disadvantaged populations.

He serves on the Secretary of Health and Human Service's National Advisory Committee on Health Promotion and Disease Prevention (Healthy People 2020) and on the Community Guide for Preventive Services Health Marketing Review. He also advises numerous social change organizations about health communication and marketing strategies, including Population Services International, Prevent Child Abuse America and the Medical Research Council in South Africa. Dr. Evans received his Bachelor of Arts in psychology and philosophy from Reed College in 1984. He went on to attain a Master of Arts and Ph.D. in cognitive science from the Johns Hopkins University in 1988 and 1991.

Robert J. Gould, Ph.D., is a behavioral scientist who has helped lead some of the nation's most successful social marketing campaigns. President and CEO of Partnership for Prevention, Dr. Gould previously served as the director of Culture/Brand Integration at Crispin Porter + Bogusky Group. From 2001 to 2007, he was a partner at Porter Novelli and Managing Director of its Washington office—the second largest operation within the firm. Dr. Gould served as leader of Porter Novelli's Health and Social Marketing practice, working on anti-tobacco accounts that included the award-winning "truth" campaign. He also worked with the American Cancer Society, the National Cancer Institute, the National Institute on Drug Abuse, the National Heart, Lung, and Blood Institute, Centers for Disease Control and Prevention, and the American Heart Association. Dr. Gould was the lead researcher in developing the now iconic Food Guide

Pyramid for the United States Department of Agriculture. In 1978, he received a Ph.D. in social psychology at the University of Maryland and graduated Phi Beta Kappa from Bucknell University in 1973.

Jeffrey C. Greene is an inventor and entrepreneur. He is co-founder and CEO of MedEncentive, which offers a unique web-based incentive system designed to control healthcare costs. Prior to MedEncentive, Mr. Greene founded and ran CompONE Services, one of the largest and most technologically advanced practice management and medical billing firms in the country.

Mr. Greene is well-known for his passionate call to improve healthcare and promote healthiness in constructive ways that draw on free-market principles, positive incentives, behavioral science, and just plain commonsense. He was a long-time instructor at the University of Oklahoma's Family Medicine Residency Program. He co-authored a text on practice management published by the American Academy of Family Physicians. Among other charitable and professional organizations, he serves on the University of Oklahoma Industrial Engineering Advisory Committee. From 2005 through 2009, Mr. Greene was selected as an Oklahoma Innovator of the Year for an unprecedented four out of five years.

Jill Griffiths is vice president of Thought Leadership, Clinical and Provider Relations for Aetna, based in Hartford, Connecticut. She is responsible for developing thought leadership campaigns to highlight Aetna's clinical leadership, provider relations programs and activities, direct to consumer programs, and other key strategic initiatives. Ms. Griffiths co-leads Aetna's health literacy initiatives with the company's chief medical officer, is co-chair of the health literacy task force for America's Health Insurance Plans, and participates on the oral health literacy advisory group for the American Dental Association.

Previously, she was vice president of business communications, where she was responsible for public relations and employee communication for Aetna's businesses. She has been assistant vice president and director of Health Public Relations for Aetna, where she handled media relations for the health business of Aetna, and directed the regional public relations managers. Ms. Griffiths joined U.S. Healthcare in January 1996 as director of public relations, after managing the U.S. Healthcare account for Foote, Cone & Belding and the Tierney Group, agencies based in Philadelphia, PA. Ms. Griffiths holds a B.A. in english literature with a minor concentration in business administration from Ursinus College and has completed continuing education courses in advertising and public relations at Villanova University.

Juli Hermanson, M.P.H., R.D., is a senior nutrition scientist at the General Mills Bell Institute of Health and Nutrition in Minneapolis. As a registered dietitian, she specializes in nutrition communications, translating nutrition science into practical advice to promote healthy eating for consumers. With over a decade of experience at General Mills, she has been involved in food regulations, marketing strategy, and communications. She currently oversees health professional outreach for the company.

Prior to her work at General Mills, she counseled nutritionally at-risk, low-income women and their families as a nutrition counselor with the Special Supplemental Food Program for Women, Infants and Children (WIC Program). She also worked as a nutrition consultant with HealthPartners' *Better Health Restaurant Challenge*, helping Twin Cities restaurants offer healthy alternatives on their menus.

Ms. Hermanson attained a Bachelor of Science degree in dietetics at Iowa State University and completed a dietetic internship at Brigham and Women's Hospital in Boston. Additionally, she holds a Master of Public Health Nutrition from the University of Minnesota, with an emphasis in Maternal and Child Health.

Charles J. Homer, M.D., M.P.H., is president and CEO of the National Initiative for Children's Healthcare Quality, an action oriented organization headquartered in Boston, MA exclusively dedicated to improving the quality of health care for children. He is an associate professor of the Department of Society, Human Development and Health at the Harvard University School of Public Health and an associate clinical professor of pediatrics at Harvard Medical School. He was a member of the third U.S. Preventive Services Task Force from 2000 to 2002 and served as chair of the American Academy of Pediatrics Steering Committee on Quality Improvement and Management from 2001-2004. He obtained his bachelor's degree from Yale University, his medical degree from the University of Pennsylvania, and a master's degree in public health from the University of North Carolina at Chapel Hill.

George Isham, M.D., M.S., is medical director and chief health officer for HealthPartners. He is responsible for quality and utilization management, chairs the Benefits Committee, and leads Partners for Better Health, a program and strategy for improving member health. Before his current position, Dr. Isham was medical director of MedCenters Health Plan in Minneapolis. In the late 1980s, he was executive director of University Health Care, an organization affiliated with the University of Wisconsin in Madison.

Dr. Isham received his Master of Science in preventive medicine/ administrative medicine at the University of Wisconsin, Madison, and his Doctor of Medicine from the University of Illinois. He completed an internship and residency in internal medicine at the University of Wisconsin Hospital and Clinics in Madison. His experience as a primary care physician included eight years at the Freeport Clinic in Freeport, Illinois, and three years as clinical assistant professor in medicine at the University of Wisconsin.

HealthPartners is a consumer-governed Minnesota health plan that formed through the 1992 affiliation of Group Health, Inc., and MedCenters Health Plan. HealthPartners is a large managed health care organization in Minnesota, representing nearly 800,000 members. Group Health, founded in 1957, is a network of staff medical and dental centers located throughout the Twin Cities. MedCenters, founded in 1972, is a network of contracted physicians serving members through affiliated medical and dental centers.

John M. Montgomery, M.D., M.P.H., is presently vice president for Professional Relations with Blue Cross Blue Shield of Florida (BCBSF). Prior to his present appointment, he was managing medical director for Professional Affairs and Quality also with BCBSF. Prior to joining BCBSF, Dr. Montgomery served as the Medicare medical director for the State of Florida. He served as the director of Health Services and medical epidemiologist for the Duval County Health Department, assistant professor of Community Health and Family Medicine at the University of Florida, and interim director of the Volusia County Health Department.

Dr. Montgomery is actively involved in all levels of organized medicine including the American College of Physician Executives, American Academy of Family Physicians, the American Medical Association, and Florida Medical Association. He is immediate past president of the Duval County Medical Society and serves on the board of the Florida Division of the American Cancer Society.

He received his B.A. from Brown University, his Master of Public Health from the Yale University School of Medicine, and his medical degree from Brown University School of Medicine. He completed his family practice internship and residency at Naval Hospital Jacksonville, and is board certified in family practice and a fellow of the American Academy of Family Physicians. Dr. Montgomery is a certified physician executive, as well as a certified health insurance executive, and has extensive experience in health care administration, managed care, strategic planning, and public health.

Linda Neuhauser, Dr.P.H., M.P.H., is a clinical professor in the Division of Community Health and Human Development at University of California (UC), Berkeley, School of Public Health. Her research and teaching are focused on health literacy and the effectiveness of collaboratively designed communication and community health initiatives. She is co-principal investigator of the UC Berkeley Health Research for Action center, which uses participatory research methods to create and test statewide health communication that is relevant to the literacy, language, cultural, and accessibility needs of the intended users. The resources cover a broad range of topics including: health care navigation, parenting, fall prevention, care-giving, disabilities, and wellness, and have reached over 30 million households in the United States and overseas.

Dr. Neuhauser also heads the risk communication and media relations component of the UC Berkeley Center for Infectious Disease Preparedness, and serves on national task forces in the areas of communication, internet health, and bio-defense preparedness. She participated in the Surgeon General's Workshop on Health Literacy, and was a member of the U.S. Food and Drug Administration's Risk Communication Advisory Committee. Previously, she served as a health officer in the U.S. Department of State in West and Central Africa. She holds Dr.P.H. and M.P.H. degrees from the UC Berkeley School of Public Health.

Conrad Person is director of Corporate Contributions at Johnson & Johnson, a position he has assumed since 1998. Mr. Person's responsibilities include overseeing Johnson & Johnson's philanthropy portfolio in Sub-Saharan Africa, with an emphasis on saving and improving the lives of women and children; building health care capacity, primarily through education; and preventing diseases and reducing stigma associated with disease. He also manages the Head Start-Johnson & Johnson Management Fellows Program, an executive training program for Head Start directors held annually at the UCLA Anderson School of Management.

Mr. Person is an expert in humanitarian product donations and served as board chair of the Partnership for Quality Medical Donations, a non-profit membership association for pharmaceutical and medical device manufacturers dedicated to raising the standards for medical donations worldwide. He was the founding board chair of the Association for Corporate Contributions Professionals, an organization devoted to enhancing the impact of corporate giving programs through professional development. Mr. Person is a graduate of Princeton University and has more than 25 years of manufacturing and human resources experience in the medical device and pharmaceutical industries.

Scott C. Ratzan, M.D., M.P.A., M.A., is vice president of Global Health at Johnson & Johnson, and editor-in-chief of the *Journal of Health Communication: International Perspectives*. Previously, he was a senior technical adviser in the Bureau of Global Health at the U.S. Agency for International Development. He also has served on expert committees for the World Health Organization, American Medical Association, and Institute of Medicine, as well as other U.S. government agencies.

Following a decade in Boston (1988-1998) in academia as founder and director of the Emerson-Tufts Program in Health Communication, a joint master's degree program between Emerson College and Tufts University School of Medicine, Dr. Ratzan moved to Washington focusing on health policy and communication. He continues to maintain faculty appointments at Yale University School of Medicine, Tufts University School of Medicine, and George Washington University Medical Center, as well as the College of Europe in Belgium. Dr. Ratzan received his M.D. from the University of Southern California, M.P.A. from the John F. Kennedy School of Government at Harvard University, and M.A. from Emerson College.

Arnold Saperstein, M.D., is the president and CEO of MetroPlus Health Plan in New York City. He began his career in managed care in 1992, and then joined MetroPlus Health Plan in 1995 initially as chief medical officer and then as president and CEO since 2006. He has focused a major portion of his career in developing programs to ensure the highest quality of care delivery to the members of his plan. Under his guidance, MetroPlus was named the highest scoring plan for quality and overall customer satisfaction in New York City for three years in a row.

Dr. Saperstein received his medical degree from the New York University School of Medicine, and completed a residency in internal medicine and a fellowship in endocrinology at the New York University Medical Center programs. He has continued to practice on a weekly basis in the field of endocrinology at Bellevue Hospital.

RADM Penelope Slade-Sawyer, P.T., M.S.W., is Deputy Assistant Secretary for Health, Disease Prevention and Health Promotion, and director of the Office of Disease Prevention and Health Promotion (ODPHP), Office of Public Health and Science, in the U.S. Department of Health and Human Services (HHS). She is also a commissioned corps officer in the U.S. Public Health Service.

As the Deputy Assistant Secretary for Health, RADM Slade-Sawyer is responsible for strengthening the disease prevention and health promotion priorities of the Department within the collaborative framework of the HHS agencies. She is a senior health advisor to the Assistant Secretary of Health and to the Secretary of HHS. RADM Slade-Sawyer leads the ODPHP in coordinating three key initiatives for HHS: Healthy People 2010, the Dietary Guidelines for Americans, and the 2008 Physical Activity Guidelines for Americans. Together, these efforts focus both on preventing disease by addressing major risk factors (such as physical inactivity and poor nutrition) and on reducing the burden of disease through appropriate health screenings and prevention of secondary conditions.

Prior to her Deputy Assistant Secretary appointment, RADM Slade-Sawyer served as a senior public health advisor in the Immediate Office of the Assistant Secretary for Health. Before joining the Office of Public Health and Science, RADM Slade-Sawyer activated and led the Physical Rehabilitation Department at the Federal Medical Center, Butner, North Carolina, as the Chief of Physical Rehabilitation. RADM Slade-Sawyer earned a degree in physical therapy and a master's degree in social work from the University of North Carolina at Chapel Hill.

Appendix C

Commissioned Paper

Integrating Health Literacy into Primary and Secondary Prevention Strategies

Scott C. Ratzan, M.D., M.P.A., M.A.
Vice President, Global Health, Johnson & Johnson
and
Editor-in-Chief, Journal of Health Communication: International Perspectives

September 15, 2009
Institute of Medicine Roundtable on Health Literacy
Washington, DC

ACKNOWLEDGMENTS

Wendy Meltzer, M.P.H., Managing Editor of the *Journal of Health Communication* provided expert research and editing to this paper. Ruth Parker, M.D., and Ken Moritsugu, M.D., also provided expertise and review to earlier versions of this draft.

Disclaimer: The ideas presented here are the author's only and do not represent the positions of Johnson & Johnson.

INTEGRATING HEALTH LITERACY INTO PRIMARY AND SECONDARY PREVENTION STRATEGIES

Leaders from around the world recently endorsed a need for health literacy action at governmental levels. Culminating a year of the United Nations Economic and Social Council focusing on "Implementing the internationally agreed goals and commitments in regard to global public health," Ministers agreed in a declaration that: "We stress that health literacy is an important factor in ensuring significant health outcomes and in this regard call for the development of appropriate action plans to promote health literacy" (July 9, 2009).

In addition to dialogue at the United Nations, the European Union, OECD, United States, China, United Kingdom, and other countries have begun to address health literacy. In the United States, legislation has been introduced in the last Congress with a Senate Bill (National Health Literacy Act of 2007 (S. 2424)). HHS included health literacy as a Healthy People 2010 objective; and agencies including AHRQ, FDA, and CDC have some references to health literacy. Currently, health reform legislation includes references with health literacy and 12 states are developing legislation and/or coalitions related to health literacy.

Health literacy is a critically important, but often overlooked, determinant of health. Low health literacy skills are associated with less healthy choices, riskier behaviors, poorer health, more hospitalizations and higher healthcare costs (IOM, 2004).

> Health literacy is *"the capacity to obtain, interpret and understand basic health information and services and the competence to use such information and services to enhance health."* (IOM, 2004; Ratzan and Parker, 2000)

The purpose of this paper is to describe ways that health literacy can be effectively integrated into primary and secondary prevention in the United States. The most obvious strategy is to leverage any existing programs in health care and public health, and to reform health policy. There are many issues and challenges, but also many potential entry points, from direct to the individual to messages for broader society, through ethical health communication. Illustrative ideas are presented for policy-making consideration at the multiple levels—institutional, community, national and regional—that shape the social and structural factors which advance public health. This paper also presents a galvanizing opportunity to advance health literacy in relation to primary and secondary prevention to serve as a provocative challenge for the IOM Roundtable.

HISTORY AND BACKGROUND—CONCEPTUAL CONSTRUCTS

Winslow's definition of public health put forth 90 years ago serves as a benchmark of what we are trying to accomplish with health literacy:

Public health is the science and art of preventing disease, prolonging life and promoting physical health and efficacy through organized community efforts for the sanitation of the environment, the control of communicable infections, the education of the individual in personal hygiene, the organization of medical and nursing services for the early diagnosis and preventive treatment of disease, and the development of social machinery which will ensure every individual in the community a standard of living adequate for the maintenance of health; so organizing these benefits in such a fashion as to enable every citizen to realize his birthright and longevity. (Winslow, 1920)

Further, the IOM definition put forth in the *Future of Public Health*, (now over 20 years old) defined the mission of public health as "fulfilling society's interest in assuring conditions in which people can be healthy" (IOM, 1988). Health literacy fits these 20th century ideals, with an opportune time for 21st century interventions.

Linking the ideas of prevention and wellness with health literacy may seem obvious, but do not seem to have been a focus of research. Historically, there has been political dialogue on the topic. The 1951 President's Commission on the Health Needs of the Nation, formed by President Truman to provide recommendations about how to meet the nation's immediate and long-term health care requirements, published a landmark work touching on issues of health promotion (as opposed to disease treatment) entitled the Magnuson Report (named for the Commission's chairman, Dr. Paul A. Magnuson). It was holistic in that it concluded that if a person's social environment involved a lack of basic security such as food, shelter, or employment, the achievement of positive health (and wellness) was much more difficult than if these were not a source of stress. This suggested that social capital that included a network of supportive social and cultural institutions were necessary to support the individual in his quest to achieve high level wellness. Further, in 1961, Halbert Dunn introduced the idea of high-level wellness as "an integrated method of functioning which is oriented toward maximizing the potential of which the individual is capable. It requires that the individual maintain a continuum of balance a purposeful direction within the environment where he is functioning" (Dunn, 1961; Ratzan, 2009).

Years later, the health field model became the basis of the IOM (1997) report titled *Improving Health in the Community: A Role for Performance Monitoring*. The model, as described by Evans and Stoddart (1994), suggested multiple determinants of health in a dynamic relationship, linking the social environment, physical environment, genetic endowment, an individual's behavioral and biologic responses, disease, health care, health and function, well-being, and prosperity. This "field" model builds on the earlier health field framework of Blum and Lalonde (see also Collins, 1995; Hancock, 1993; Mustard and Frank, 1991). This model has been advanced recently as a "21st century field model" (Ratzan et al., 2000).

While it is beyond the scope of this article to address comprehensive theoretical developments for advancing health, the field model demonstrates the relationships between the elements that contribute to health. Health literacy can be the most important contributor to health as it presents an opportunity for health literacy application in addressing the necessary skills and abilities in synch with the demands and complexity of the system. Improving a population's health literacy promotes health and can prevent a great amount of disease and disability. Understanding what you need to do to "be healthy" and building systems of care and services that are navigable and accessible are foundational and fundamental for improving population health. Efforts to enhance population health literacy, and primary and secondary prevention are intricately linked and together create a double helix as a foundation for health reform. Such a health literacy helix serves as the fabric for improving health in America as it translates primary and secondary prevention into (1) what we need to know and do to stay healthy, and (2) detecting and treating disease early to get better and/or live with disease. In this paper, relevant findings from health literacy research help develop a framework for action, with specific recommendations for policymakers.

RELEVANT LESSONS FROM HEALTH LITERACY RESEARCH

The lack of health literacy in the U.S. population has been well-documented in the 2004 IOM report, *Health Literacy: A Prescription to End Confusion*. Only 12 percent of adults have proficient health literacy. According to the NAAL, nearly 9 out of 10 American adults lack the skills needed to take care of their own health, and most do not know how to prevent disease. This is concerning for the health of most Americans but also for the burden it places on our health care system. Limited health literacy is estimated to cost the nation between $100 and $200 billion a year (Vernon et al., 2007). Today, chronic diseases—such as cancer, diabetes, and heart disease—are among the most prevalent, costly, and preventable of all health problems. Health literacy is at the center of both preventing chronic disease and adhering to treatment plans once diagnosed. Furthermore, obesity related conditions account for 9.1 percent of medical spending or $147 billion—extra expenses of diabetes and other ailments that are more common in an overweight population could be addressed with health literacy interventions. This can translate into significant savings as medical spending averages $1,400 more a year for an obese person than for someone of normal weight (Finkelstein et al., 2009).

There have been over 1,000 studies on health literacy that address prevalence, outcomes, and costs to society and the individual (Rudd, 2006). The IOM and AHRQ have also comprehensively reviewed the literature in the last 5 years on health literacy and health outcomes and "concluded that limited health literacy is negatively associated with the use of preventive services like mammograms or flu shots; management of chronic conditions such as diabetes, high blood pressure, asthma, and HIV/AIDS; and self-reported health" (Berkman et al., 2004; IOM, 2004). Studies have also linked limited health literacy to misunderstanding of prescription medication instructions, medication errors, poor comprehension of nutrition labels, and mortality (Baker et al., 2008; Davis et al., 2006a, 2006b; Rothman et al., 2006; Wolf et al., 2006).

Finally, as much as 88 percent of adults have difficulty with the way health information is currently presented and most do not have the ability to recognize and understand risk, sort through conflicting information, act upon information, and navigate our frequently complex health systems (WHCA, 2009). Given the importance for individuals to interpret and act upon critical public health alerts, along with a system that needs to simplify and clarify communication to address emerging threats, a lack of health literacy increases the risk for the entire population during acute health crises, such as the 2009 novel H1N1 pandemic.

Today, we have the knowledge to begin to address health literacy with interventions. Health literacy has been defined, plausible models of antecedent factors and causes elucidated, and now we are ready to develop and test intervention strategies, implement policies and communication, and evaluate and refine those interventions. Health literacy strategies need to be woven into prevention efforts at all levels, and building one's health literacy should be thought of as a lifelong process. Even simple, small initiatives and interventions can dramatically improve health literacy and outcomes and associated costs.

LINKING HEALTH LITERACY AND PREVENTION

Preventive care . . . is one of the best ways to keep our people healthy and our costs under control. Remarks of President Barack Obama—as prepared for delivery address to Joint Session of Congress, February 24, 2009.

While ethical premises and age old adages suggest prevention of disease as preferential to treatment, reducing risk and promoting healthful behaviors have not been the foundation for the U.S. health system.

Primary prevention programs and strategies that provide access to health information that is clear, easy-to-understand and meaningful to the individual and that address common risk factors for chronic disease such as obesity, physical inactivity, and blood pressure control could be addressed through a health literacy prism. Such programs help individuals identify modifiable risk and protective factors for diseases/disorders/injuries; and assess risk, including genetic susceptibility.

Secondary prevention seeks to stop or slow down existing disease and its effects through early detection and appropriate treatment. This would include efforts such as screening and management of diabetes, heart or respiratory diseases or early detection of cancer. Even seemingly highly educated patients can have trouble understanding basic health information. We need to build bridges between what we as health professionals know, and what our patients understand.

In looking at the recent literature on health literacy and prevention, relatively few studies examined low health literacy and its effect on primary prevention efforts that target risk factors for chronic disease (such as obesity, blood pressure) and few studies describe health literacy interventions in this specific area. Yet, there are many studies that measure and validate the malleable lifestyle factors that serve as variables in the Field Model and conceptual underpinning of health literacy. For example, recent large studies published in the Archives of Internal Medicine (Jiao et al., 2009; Mozaffarian et al., 2009) identified five lifestyle factors as contributors to pancreatic cancer and diabetes. These five factors alone accounted for a 58 percent reduction in risk of developing pancreatic cancer, and attributability for diabetes incidence in 90 percent of new cases. These 5 variables include smoking, alcohol use, diet, body mass index, and physical activity. Other studies have suggested that adding variables such as fasting blood sugar, blood pressure, cholesterol levels, immunization(s) and other areas (cancer screening) also could translate into better health outcomes and reduced health costs.

Given the plethora of evidence from a variety of fields (e.g., communication, public health, medicine, etc.) an evidence-informed approach to primary and secondary prevention efforts could be advanced within these domains (*Journal of Health Communication*, 2006). In 2006, U.S. Surgeon General Ken Moritsugu summed this up well in a speech on disparities; "more research is needed, but there is already enough good information that we can use to make practical improvements in health literacy."

Where to Start—The Model

Health literacy can be achieved through the lens of a simple model (Figure C-1): when individuals skills and ability are appropriately aligned

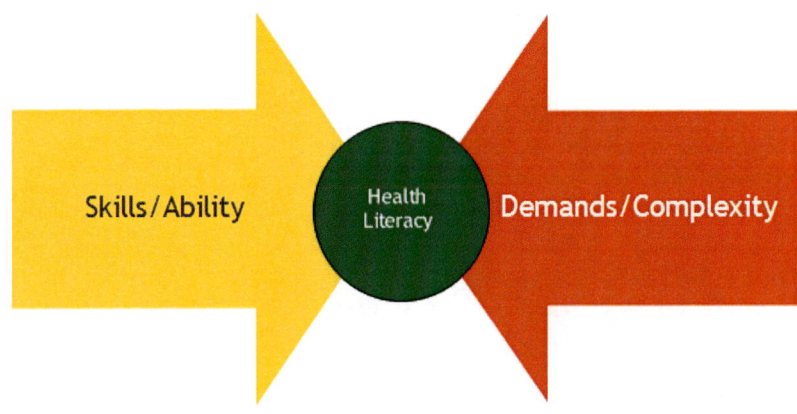

FIGURE C-1 Health literacy framework.
SOURCE: Parker, 2009.

with system demands and complexity (IOM, 2004; WHCA, 2009). Skills are cognitive (knowledge), behavioral (functional), and advocatory (pro-active).

Health literacy occurs when the skills and ability of those requiring health information and services are aligned with the demand and complexity of information and services. While we continue to support efforts to improve the skills and ability of all through educational efforts, we intervene by improving the navigability and understandability of that which is required for better health. The model indicates that the skills and ability of individuals (yellow) slow one down as they approach tasks, as many lack the skills to understand and do what they need to do for health. However, it is the demands and complexity of health information and task (red) that stop many from being able to do what they need to do for health. Interventions to simplify and improve the demands and complexity are the top priority for action, and we must work to systematically make health more understandable and services more navigable for patients. To be "patient centered" and to improve quality, the alignment of skills and ability with the demands and complexity of essential tasks advances a health literate populace (green).

Kickbusch and Maag (2008) have suggested 6 principal domains that affect how people make daily decisions that affect their health: the health care system, home, the community, the workplace, the market place (i.e., the media) and the political arena. To create a road map to strengthen health literacy in the United States in the areas of primary and secondary prevention, this paper is organized by clustering these domains into three areas: (1) prevention within the health care system, (2) educational system, home community and workplace, and (3) media and new technology. For each, we look at how efforts can work simultaneously to systematically address the demand and complexity of tasks and advance the population's skills to obtain, process and turn good information into action. Further, to best advance health literacy with primary prevention in these areas, a parsimonious idea is first presented: a "scorecard" that could possibly reflect an individual or population's level of alignment of predetermined goals and actual level of health achievements. Such "scorecards" could be proxies for reflecting what an individual or population understands and sets as their health goals, and how close they are to actually achieving these goals.

A Simple (Parsimonious), But Big Idea

On the area of measuring health, there have been ideas to develop some sort of galvanizing index that captures health and wellness. In the last decade the IOM has had two committees addressing this: Leading Health Indicators for Healthy People 2010 (final report in 1999) and State of the USA (final report in 2009).[1] The recommendations from these IOM committee reports offered ideas and policy directions; at this point, neither have been instituted.

The "new" idea here is to develop a measureable health literacy scorecard. Such a scorecard could add significant value in spurring action on health literacy that could facilitate individual and system monitoring of health literacy. The individual scorecard would identify a limited number of key health indicators that are associated with a healthy physical and mental state. A composite score could include fasting blood sugar (diabetes), body mass index (obesity), cholesterol (cardiovascular disease), blood pressure (hypertension), smoking/tobacco use (cancer and CVD), immunizations (vaccine preventable disease), and cancer screenings (age and gender specific). Individuals could get a "score" and rate themselves against a standard that could have predictive value for age and disease probability. The score could be developed with formative research that could be presented in the form of a grade A-F, percentile, gradation, color scheme, all-or-none or other easy-to-understand and galvanizing level for action (Nolan and Berwick, 2006). The challenge here will be to ensure that the variables selected could be addressed with interventions to build

---

[1] The author served on the IOM Leading Health Indicator Committee and suggested a potential framework that would address health and wellness entitled POISE "a balance— physical, occupational, intellectual, social/spiritual and emotional approaches" as dimensions for health. While this was discussed as a framework for the committee, it principally became a theoretical construct in health communication joining other wellness-related contexts with health communication teacher-scholars ontology.

health literacy (e.g., communication, policy and system engineering) so that the nexus of this score could be a reflection of the skills and ability of the individual and the demands and complexity of the system that foster a better "score." These could be packaged in a way such that a "personal" health score could give people a general idea of what these mean, dialogue points to discuss with their physician and ample interest to get their "score" both on the individual measures and the composite, into a range that would translate into better health (and possibly lower costs and health spending [e.g., premiums]). Of course, as this is science and evidence based, health literate people would feel better, be sick less, be more productive at work and home and strengthen the new "personalized population health" (with a double helix of health literacy and prevention).

These scorecards and variable could be developed and updated on a national level with appropriate evidence and expertise from multistakeholders—pediatric health literacy chaired by AAP, maternal health literacy by ACOG, secondary prevention for people with diabetes by ADA, (see commissioned paper appendix for an example on the D5) etc., as well as a list suggested by IOM selected from the preventive services task force recommendations and other evidence/consensus based approaches. This scorecard could be viewed as a reflection of personal or population skills to understand evidence based goals and the degree of alignment health systems have to make these goals understandable, navigable, and accessible to those seeking them. Health literacy "scorecards" thus would reflect the alignment of skills and task demands and complexity. Additionally, such a scorecard or composite index at multiple levels could reflect the health literacy status of individuals and groups to further inform and motivate health communication campaigns, programs and resources (Ratzan, 2009; WHCA, 2009).

Furthermore, the scorecard could be tailored, endorsed and diffused in the three areas discussed in the next section of this paper.

Domain One:
Prevention and Health Literacy Within the Healthcare System

The health care system has a major role in developing individual and population health literacy skills. The influence of the health care system can be seen through the services it provides, the way its workers are trained and interact with individuals, the ease of navigation for patients, and the way the system supports an individual's ability to get the information he or she needs and acts upon it in an appropriate manner. The health care system can foster (and hinder) obtaining information and services for individuals with all levels of health literacy skills. A large part of prevention lies in the responsibilities of the health care system and health professionals to communicate in such a way so that those we serve, can hear, understand, embrace, and act upon the science/evidence-based professional advice provided for them, so they can make better health decisions. This becomes even more critical when addressing prevention of chronic diseases.

The health system can be a cornerstone with interventions that promote healthful behaviors with the provision of health information addressing common risk factors for chronic disease such as diet, physical inactivity and blood pressure control and interventions that help patients (and the public) understand how to manage their existing disease and its effects through early detection and appropriate treatment.

"The greatest opportunities for reducing health disparities are in empowering individuals and changing the health system to meet their needs" (HHS, 2000). As Moritsugu stated "without clear communication and easier access to services, we can't expect people to adopt the health behaviors and take the actions we champion . . . the promises of medical research, health information technology, and advances in health care delivery cannot be realized without also addressing health literacy. Limited health literacy is not an individual deficit but a systematic problem that should be addressed by ensuring that health care and health information systems are aligned with the needs of the public" (Moritsugu, 2006).

Understanding Health Information

It can be difficult for anyone, no matter the literacy skills, to remember instructions or read a label when sick. Health care professionals, public health officials, and the media often present information in ways that make information and services more difficult to understand and use than they need to be. Some of these elusive skills are basic: such as reading, writing, and numeracy, and the ability to communicate and question. Even for people with basic health literacy, patient education brochures, informed consent forms, notices of privacy protection, patient bills of rights, and labels on medications can be too complex (previous IOM reports). Ineffective communication between health providers and patients can result in medical errors due to misunderstandings about medications and instructions.

A groundbreaking achievement of the IOM health literacy report was the acknowledgement that the epidemic of poor health literacy actually reflects a problem in the way health information is communicated to people what they must do to take care of their health. This framing of health literacy shifts the focus from improving individual patient health literacy skills to encouraging broader system change. Are essential tasks for promoting, protecting, and managing health clearly defined, described, and communicated so that they are understandable and action-able? Is the use of technical jargon in both written and spoken language minimized? The overall objective of health literacy is to align the required tasks and demands with the skills and ability of patients and consumers. At present we have significant misalignment.

At all levels of preventive care, health materials that are easier to read along with meaningful personal interactions with healthcare pro-viders can advance understanding. Patients struggle to articulate what is wrong with them and doctors struggle equally to convey information that is understandable. Often, the very same patients with limited health literacy are also those individuals and groups without access to providers. Whereas in the past, health management was left to the physician, many health systems now encourage individuals to take more responsibility for their own health. To make appropriate "self-management" decisions, people must locate health information, evaluate the information for cred-ibility and quality, and analyze risks and benefits. Furthermore, people must be able to understand the available medical information, ask perti-nent questions and express health concerns clearly by describing symp-toms in ways the providers can understand (IOM, 2004).

Patient education is an important focus for prevention of costly hos-pital readmissions. Patients are prescribed medications, but without the ability to comprehend the instructions, they make frequent errors or do not adhere correctly to important regimens. In addition there is a dif-ference between adherence (patient reports of following regimen) and concordance (clinician-patient agreement regarding regimen). A lack of functional health literacy has been found to impair patient's understand-ing in both written and oral communication with caregivers (Schillinger, 2006). To advance better understanding, health literate disease manage-ment programs could be designed for patients with varying literacy skills.

Ease of Use/Navigation of the Health System

It is critical for patients to understand their own health system and its demands and requirements for primary and secondary prevention. A recent national survey of older adults who receive Medicare measured familiarity with health insurance terminology and proficiency with using the Medicare program. They found that the overall level of health insur-ance literacy among this population was low to moderate, with the oldest adults with poorer health and lower income levels at the lower end of that spectrum of literacy (McCormack et al., 2009). There are assessment tools to evaluate the extent to which a health service meets the needs of patients with limited health literacy skills. One example, applied to a pharmacy setting, was found to be a vital component of evaluating patient understanding of medications and adherence to prescribed regimens. Also, the tool raised pharmacy staff awareness of health literacy issues and detected barriers that may have prevented individuals with limited literacy skills from accessing, comprehending, and using health information and services provided by the organization (Jacobson, 2008).

The health care system needs to be more proactive and take responsibility to meet the needs of the people it serves. Reducing the health literacy demands placed on individuals by such actions as modifying consent processes (Sudore et al., 2009); redesigning forms in advance to meet low literacy needs (Sudore et al., 2007); and emphasizing the importance of health literacy training for health care professionals will be steps toward this goal.

Training Providers in Communication

Health systems and the tasks they require of patients must continue to be simplified and physicians and other providers need to be prepared to handle the communication needs of growingly diverse patient populations, educating providers on how best to communicate with patients with widely divergent health literacy (Berkman et al., 2004). Health professionals and administrators must closely examine how patients engage their clinics and affiliated organizations, and work toward a truly patient-centered process.

Treating low health literacy as a "universal precaution" and training health providers, schools, and local community organizations in high risk areas in health communication "best practices" as a rule (Paasche-Orlow et al., 2006), and employing strategies to improve patient education and clinician-patient communication approaches benefit all patients, and harm none (Pignone et al., 2005). If the content and delivery of essential patient information is standardized (if not regulated) patients will be able to better form certain expectations of their health care experience.

Paasche-Orlow et al. (2006) suggest many ways that the health system can address limited literacy. Promoting better interactions between patients and providers, reorganizing, streamlining health care delivery; embracing a 21st-century field model approach with a community level and ecological perspective that acknowledges the various factors influencing health and health care for those with limited literacy. Each of these factors affects how we communicate, understand, and respond to health information.

As stated in an AHRQ review of health literacy, "it is often assumed that improved written communication can improve health outcomes. However, research suggests that improving information delivery alone may not mitigate the observed relationship between low literacy and poor health. Addressing other important factors, such as self-efficacy, self-care, trust, or satisfaction, may increase our understanding of effective strategies for addressing poor health outcomes" (Berkman et al., 2004). For example, a recent study shows that providing patients with literacy-appropriate information, coupled with counseling is effective for improving self management of diabetes (Wallace et al., 2009). This suggests the types of strategies we might work toward for prevention and ongoing support for chronic disease (see commissioned paper appendix).

Domain Two:
Educational System, Home, Community, and Workplace

We are increasingly challenged to make sound health decisions in the context of everyday life. As we read and interpret product labels and warnings; make lifestyle choices regarding eating, activity, smoking and drugs; evaluate the safety of chemicals in products we buy, find and interpret trustworthy health information on the Internet, we use our health literacy skills. Such everyday demands require individuals to be able to assess their current health and recognize the many socioeconomic factors and cultural values that influence it. For all this they need to have health literacy competencies and learned abilities that allow them to take responsibility for their own and their family's (and, where necessary, their community's) health (Kickbusch and Maag, 2008).

Health literacy is linked across sectors. At present, few healthcare professionals receive formal training in communication, particularly in working with people with limited literacy. In recent years, the National Board of Medical Examiners has added a one-day exam for all medical students that includes an assessment of communication and interpersonal skills. However, the clinical skills test does not specifically address how limited health literacy affects interactions with patients. And most healthcare professionals already in practice have not had formal training in improving communication skills. A growing number of continuing medical education courses in health literacy are available. The American Medical Association and the federal Health Resources and Services Administration both have training available for professionals who provide healthcare services. Imagine if every medical student, resident and physician were taught to present cases and ensure patients understood their prevention needs and actions as a standardized part of clinical presentations. The Subjective, Objective, Assessment, and Plan could add a P for "Prevention" to become SOAPP. If this intervention/measure were added, with commensurate measurement and reimbursement (short and long term) to attain such a quality standard, there might be some movement that would match policy with practice.

Increasing patient skills across the lifespan through all levels of the education system is critical. School-age children should be taught about nutrition, hygiene, vaccinations and common symptoms/illness as part of their elementary curriculum; prevention and screening for cancer screening information could be added (breast self examinations, testicular examinations, annual pap smears) to reproductive health classes as children age to adolescents. Teaching accurate, standards-based, culturally and developmentally appropriate health and science education should start in early childhood education and continue through the university level. We also need to support and expand local efforts to provide adult education, English language instruction, and health information services in the community (see commissioned paper appendix).

With the increase in the number of people living with chronic disease, we are shifting toward a model of the medical home. In this model, families take on a greater burden in health care. People with chronic diseases have more health literacy demands including the need for self management, coordinating care with multiple providers, managing multiple lifelong prescription medications, yet often have fewer health literacy skills. We need to equip families and communities with self care strategies. Low caregiver literacy is common and is associated with poor preventive care behaviors and poor child health outcomes. Culturally appropriate and important health information is critical to allow families to engage in health promotion, prevention, and self care activities. Family caregivers could be a key component to achieving a better health outcome, and their health literacy must also be considered when they receive health information along with the patient (Bevan and Pecchioni, 2008). "Future research should aim to ameliorate literacy-associated child health disparities" (Sanders et al., 2009).

Health literacy in the workplace can lead to accident prevention as well as the avoidance of industrial or occupational diseases. Health-promoting work environments go further and can address lifestyle choices and stress factors, including an adequate work–life balance. Much can be done in this area to promote an infrastructure that facilitates and supports access to understandable and actionable health information and services. As the current health insurance system is largely employment based, this puts employers in the role of shaping the health information and services available to Americans. There is value in a "health literate workforce." Employers are positioned to know the skills of their workforce and can use this knowledge about their employees to create on-site programs that build employees' health literacy skills and help insurance companies and health information providers create employee-friendly information and services. They can provide training for employees to improve their health information seeking and decision-making skills. Prioritizing wellness initiatives and developing policies that improve health information and services for employees and their families ultimately benefits both the employer and employee with fewer days lost to sick leave. Here is another area where a "Health Literacy Scorecard" can be introduced as a tool for advancing wellness and prevention through education. Further, over time, both the health literacy status, health outcomes, productivity and other financial variables could be collected to reflect the health literacy status of the workforce and their dependents.

There are many ideas and emphases in primary and secondary prevention with evidence based suggestions for health awareness, behavior change, employee engagement and supportive environments. Ideally, demonstration of health outcomes (including productivity, absenteeism vs. presenteeism, etc.) could be coupled with economic incentives to advance a health literate workforce. As there is increasing dialogue about an infectious disease outbreak such as H1N1, reaching people at the workplace and in their workplace networks with a health literate approach has increased salience and timeliness.

Domain Three:
Media and New Technology

Technology is evolving into a mechanism by which many people access and research health issues. Interventions need to be developed to reach people through communication technology. Programs are in place to use text-messaging to deliver prenatal care messages (i.e., vaccinations, folic acid supplementation, etc.) and states are piloting programs to use technology to reach their underserved populations (see commissioned paper appendix).

The media presents a health information marketplace within communities that shapes people's perceptions, behaviors, and choices. Notices of recalls, imminent pandemics, even labeling changes on medications, are first experienced via multiple media channels and through family and friends. Yet most individuals do not have the ability to recognize and understand risk and sort through conflicting information, so what are they to make of news reports that lack guidance on how they are to act upon the given information? A 2008 survey by the Missouri School of Journalism found that only 18 percent of journalists surveyed had specialized training in health reporting and 50 percent were not familiar with health literacy (Smith, 2008). Yet, this is who a large part of the population relies upon for health information. Adults at all levels of health literacy use multiple sources to obtain health information. But, for all levels of health literacy, no single type of print material was as important as non-print sources, such as radio or television. Adults at the below basic level of literacy were the least likely to use any written material to obtain information on health topics. At the below basic level, 43 percent used written information infrequently (HHS, 2008).

Within the media marketplace, effective communication strategies frame issues for the public of what they should think about. Communicators, public health advocates, educators, promoters, and journalists can use a wide range of technologies, media, and social marketing approaches to get independent evidence-based information to stand out and help shape people's perceptions, choices and behaviors.

Credible, reliable, accessible and understandable and actionable information is needed so that individuals can select, modify and/or avoid risky behaviors related to lifestyle choices, mental well-being, the control of infectious diseases, and environmental threats to health. Such interventions can help raise people's understanding of risks and strengthen their abilities to make healthy choices. The challenge in designing effective and understandable health communication is to determine the optimal context, channels and content which reflect the realities of people's everyday lives, situations and communication practices (IOM, 2003). The viewpoints and experiences of the targeted population need to be included in the design, implementation and evaluation of all interventions (IOM, 2004).

The Foundation: Policy and the Political Arena

Policies shape the institutional, community, and structural factors which determine health literacy and health. Active citizens can "speak-up" when institutional, community, and governmental policies and structures need to be changed. "Political" health literacy competencies include advocacy skills that promote policy change, informed voting behavior in the political arena, knowledge of health rights, and participation in civil society such as community, patient and health organizations. The economic realities are also with us; and as the hard policy choices are made, these must be part of the calculus. An informed and involved populace is critical in developing and implementing these policies. In research, practice, and policy there must be shared and integrated responsibility and involvement, with the person at the center.

CONCLUSION

Strategies to provide understandable information about realistic, achievable options to obtain optimal health that can be implemented at home, work, and in the greater community require practical supports at the individual and community level to overcome barriers. Ideally, a solid foundation of health literacy would prevent disease, but it must be acknowledged that a large part of our population is already dealing with the effects of chronic disease (e.g., diabetes) and close attention must be paid to developing strategies that stop or slow down existing disease and its effects through early detection and appropriate treatment.

Real health reform must move toward prevention as a goal while still remaining prepared for appropriate intensive and specialty care. The trend is toward a medical home where decisions are shared and negotiated by all parties in health care, with the interests of the patient and families in the center.

One of the key ideas articulated in this paper that has not been fundamentally addressed in prior dialogues or publications is the idea of a health literacy scorecard. As the world is developing a greater interest in advancing health and wellness and preventing disease, we need measures of what people need to know and do—individually at work and at home, in the community, and as citizens. A health literacy scorecard can help us aspire to making the grade with our actions in disease prevention. Such an approach would be a new way of assessing societal progress by explicitly capturing how people can view their own health, measuring progress and success at multiple levels and demonstrating the value of health in society. Rather than an economic based approach, it would be multidisciplinary and an ethical and evidence informed approach to policy-making. Finally, it also could galvanize our global institutions, national governments, civil society, the private sector, and the public to act and address issues and antecedent factors to prevent disease and advance health.

In an era of economic and political challenges, advancing health literacy is a reasonable and achievable public health goal and policy imperative in the United States. Health literacy initiatives could garner bipartisan support that can be advanced with minimal incremental investments and redirection of funding. Further, with impending challenges of pandemic flu and the challenges of educating and mobilizing a number of people with limited or poor health literacy, the exigency to advance a national health literacy action plan is timely. Moreover, most Americans are aware of this issue as they have faced problems at some point understanding health information for themselves or for a family member. And, finally, a fundamental tenet of humankind to advance health and prevent disease can drive people to action with appropriate health literate interventions that suggest what people need to know and do among a system that can simplify demands and complexity for action. By addressing "health literacy policies as fundamental for health reform" the United States can move forward and make a difference on a key underlying health care problem—and on an issue that resonates with virtually everyone.

Recommendations for Action to Support Health Literacy

Recommendation 1

Relevant agencies should develop, test and implement health communication approaches to advance wellness and prevention so that skills and abilities of the population can be aligned with the demands and complexity of the tasks required for health. Health literacy can be attained with existing and innovative communication approaches on health behaviors, as social media, tailored communication and community interventions.

Recommendation 2

The U.S. government should set a high level health literacy agenda at the Office of the Surgeon General and/or Domestic Policy Council to convene and guide agencies to fund and create a Health Literacy P-scorecard (or a variety of scorecards based upon demographic and psychographic variables) in each state at a minimum to meet basic prevention and wellness awareness and behaviors such as the population knowledge and skills and a system that supports attainment of the prevention activities.

Recommendation 3

The National Governors' Association, mayors, civic organizations, and other leading organizations could similarly address and adopt health literacy measures of their constituents that integrate primary and secondary prevention into sustainability and other social sector goals. Private public partnerships could be fostered to create demonstrations and incentives. (These could be modeled after the WHO Healthy Cities Consortium.)

Recommendation 4

HHS and public and private funders should support the development, testing, and use of simple, culturally appropriate new measures of health literacy that incorporate prevention objectives. A National Institutes of Health, IOM, or other federally supported task force should convene a consensus panel to develop the P-score or health literacy index that would initiate the development of simple (no more than 10) operational measures of primary and secondary prevention that would be relevant to age, gender, cultural, genetic, contextual, epidemiological, and geographic location.

Recommendation 5

Health care systems should develop programs that incorporate in- and outpatient approaches to simplify the demands and complexity of participants practicing prevention. Centers for Medicare and Medicaid Services (CMS) can take the lead in developing a scorecard for Medicaid and Medicare patients. Incentives could be created with health literacy strategies for better communication with seniors. Pediatric health literacy (measures and goals) could be integrated into State Children's Health Insurance Program (SCHIP) materials.

Recommendation 6

With the goal for the population to attain basic health literacy, Federal agencies responsible for addressing disparities should support the development of new quality standards that reduce the demands and complexities of the health system. The ultimate goal is to make it simple and clear what individuals must "do" to access and utilize necessary health services.

Recommendation 7

The Department of Education (at federal, state, and local levels) should develop a health literacy competency base for levels of elementary and secondary education that includes the necessary education and measurement that could be integrated into standardized testing (a score). This scorecard could be reported at various grade intervals across traditional education grades to demonstrate the health literacy knowledge skills and practice of prevention and behaviors.

Recommendation 8

Congress should adopt a healthy workplace policy for all companies that advances primary and secondary prevention that is consistent with evidence based research and strategies. An attainable scorecard with economic incentives for employees and employers such as tax credits should also be hallmark to advance adoption of health promoting behaviors

Recommendation 9

The AAMC and other accrediting boards for health professional schools and professional continuing education programs in health and related fields, including medicine, dentistry, pharmacy, social work, anthropology, nursing, public health, communication, and journalism should incorporate primary and secondary prevention health literacy into their curricula, practice, accreditations, and areas of competence.

Recommendation 10

New Activities in Comparative Effectiveness including those in development with the Federal Coordinating Committee (CMS, FDA, NIH, VA, and Defense) should integrate health literacy among the six interventions under consideration—notably the behavior change and prevention areas of interest.

COMMISSIONED PAPER APPENDIX OF CASES IN HEALTH LITERACY AND PREVENTION

DOMAIN ONE: HEALTH SYSTEMS

Case 1

Pittsburgh Regional Health Initiative—Proper use of chronic obstructive pulmonary disease medications requires many steps that are difficult to remember and do correctly. Case managers spent one hour per week for 7-8 weeks teaching patients correct use of their inhalers. In just three months, this teaching resulted in a 35 percent reduction in hospital readmissions (2008, Pittsburgh Regional Health Initiative).

Case 2

The Integrated Health Network (IHN) is a group of eight providers who serve over 200,000 uninsured and underinsured residents in St. Louis, Missouri. An IHN initiative, called the Health Education and Literacy Program, uses lay health coaches to reach uninsured and underinsured residents to empower them to take control of their health, communicate with providers, and become more confident in navigating the health delivery system. Despite barriers to healthcare among this population, including transportation access, financial obstacles, and lack of trust in the healthcare system, results of a qualitative study to determine the effectiveness of health coaches were positive. Preliminary findings revealed a significant increase in the percentage of patients who had a primary care provider after working with a health coach (from 57 percent to 81 percent). Moreover, after working with a health coach, 27 percent of chronic disease patients (up from 1 percent) are now able to discuss their self management plan.

Case 3

Chronic Disease Management Program (IOM, 2004)—Researchers and practitioners at the University of North Carolina have developed several chronic disease management programs that are designed to identify and overcome literacy-related barriers to care. The programs, which include interventions for diabetes, heart failure, chronic pain, and anticoagulation, are led by clinical pharmacist practitioners and trained health educators, who use evidence-based algorithms, a computerized patient registry, and literacy-independent teaching techniques to facilitate effective self-care and assure receipt of effective services and medications. In each area, the program organizers have systematically measured literacy as well as relevant health outcomes. For diabetes and anticoagulation, completed studies have found that these programs can offset the adverse effects of low literacy.

DOMAIN TWO: EDUCATIONAL SYSTEM, HOME, COMMUNITY, AND WORKPLACE

Case 1

Head Start Program Health Literacy Study—Parents of 20,000 children in 35 states were provided with health information and training to help them address their children's health needs. Prior to the training, 60 percent of the parents said that they did not have a health book at home to reference. Parents reported being "very confident" about caring for their sick children, yet 69 percent reported taking a child to a doctor or clinic at the first sign of illness and nearly 45 percent said they would take their child to a clinic or emergency room for a cough rather than provide care at home, even for a mild temperature of 99.5°F. Parents were given training and a medical guide to refer to when their children became sick. After training, parents using the medical guide as a first source of help jumped from 5 percent to 48 percent, indicating a better understanding and higher comfort level in dealing with common childhood illnesses. Visits to a hospital ER or clinic dropped by 58 percent and 42 percent, respectively, adding up to a potential annual savings to Medicaid of $554 per family in direct costs, or about $5.1 million annually. This translated into a 42 percent drop in the average number of days lost at work (from 6.7 to 3.8) and 29 percent drop in days children lost at school (from 13.3 to 9.5). Parents also reported feeling more confident in making health care decisions and in sharing knowledge with others in their families and communities (UCLA study).

DOMAIN THREE: MEDIA AND NEW TECHNOLOGY

Case 1

Mobile Health—The United States has the second worst infant mortality rate in the developed world. Given the challenge, later in 2009, a Text4Baby will begin with a design to leverage the more than 280 million mobile phones in the United States to deliver timely, relevant, and appropriate information to pregnant women and new mothers—particularly those in underserved populations—to improve the health of mothers and babies. Although basic maternal health information that can help reduce the chances of preterm labor and improve the health of mothers and babies is readily available in baby books and on web sites for women with access, it is not getting to the women who need it most. There is a unique opportunity for reaching lower-income women with cell phones as they are more than twice as likely to have a cell phone as broadband Internet (63 percent to 31 percent). Additionally, Hispanics and African Americans are much more likely to use their cell phones for SMS and other data services (73 percent vs. 68 percent vs. 53 percent). The Text4Baby service will send free SMS text messages to pregnant women who opt into the program with tips and information on how to take care of themselves and their babies. The evidence-based messages will answer questions like When do I need to visit a clinic?; What are signs I'm going into labor?; When should my baby be vaccinated? With formative research to confirm frequency and messages, participants will receive 3-5 messages per week based on stage of pregnancy telling what to expect, what to avoid, and what to do to help get through pregnancy safely. After the baby is born, the new mom will receive messages based on her baby's age reminding her about important check-ups, vaccinations, and tips to keep her and her baby healthy.

Case 2

Arizona's Medicaid program, the Arizona Health Care Cost Containment System (AHCCCS) is using eHealth technology to address health literacy. E-learning programs are developed specifically to address chronic conditions or other problems. The goal is to deliver education in a much more personal and culturally sensitive manner, tailoring the important content of that education to the various needs of the population and using messengers who are similar to and can relate to members of various populations. The basic website has a mission "to build health and wellness literacy in members so that they make decisions that improve their health care quality and reduce preventable health care costs through the utilization of interactive, personalized health education and health literacy competency." This website will be used to deliver many of the eHealth tools. Each beneficiary must have an e-mail address and/or document how he or she will access the Internet. If an individual does not have a way to access the Internet, then the program will take responsibility for devising a way to provide access. In this future vision, once a patient accesses his or her personal health account, the physician will be able to view the information and make sure that the patient understood the individual e-learning programs, since patient responses will be automatically uploaded to the electronic health record (EHR).

REFERENCES

Baker, D. W., M. S. Wolf, J. Feinglass, and J. A. Thompson. 2008. Health literacy, cognitive abilities, and mortality among elderly persons. *Journal of General Internal Medicine* 23(6):723-726.

Berkman, N. D., D. A. Dewalt, M. P. Pignone, S. L. Sheridan, K. N. Lohr, L. Lux, S. F. Sutton, T. Swinson, and A. J. Bonito. 2004. Literacy and health outcomes. *Evidence Report/Technology Assessment* (87):1-8.

Bevan, J. L., and L. L. Pecchioni. 2008. Understanding the impact of family caregiver cancer literacy on patient health outcomes. *Patient Education and Counseling* 71(3):356-364.

Collins, T. 1995. Models of health: Pervasive, persuasive and politically charged. *Health Promotion International* 10(4):317-324.

Davis, T. C., M. S. Wolf, P. F. Bass, M. Middlebrooks, E. Kennen, D. W. Baker, C. L. Bennett, R. Durazo-Arvizu, A. Bocchini, S. Savory, and R. M. Parker. 2006a. Low literacy impairs comprehension of prescription drug warning labels. *Journal of General Internal Medicine* 21(8):847-851.

Davis, T. C., M. S. Wolf, P. F. Bass, J. A. Thompson, H. H. Tilson, M. Neuberger, and R. M. Parker. 2006b. Literacy and misunderstanding prescription drug labels. *Annals of Internal Medicine* 145(12):887-894.

Dunn, H. L. 1961. *High-level wellness*. Arlington, VA: Beatty Press.

Evans, R. G., and G. L. Stoddart. 1994. Producing health, consuming health care. In *Why are some people healthy and others not? The determinants of health of populations*, edited by R. G. Evans, M. L. Barer, and T. R. Marmor. New York: Aldine de Gruyter.

Finkelstein, E. A., J. G. Trogdon, J. W. Cohen, and W. Dietz. 2009. Annual medical spending attributable to obesity: Payer-and service-specific estimates. *Health Affairs* 28(5): w822-w831.

Hancock, T. 1993. Health, human development and the community ecosystem: Three ecological models. *Health Promotion International* 8(1):41-47.

HHS (Department of Health and Human Services). 2000. *Healthy people 2010. 2nd ed. With understanding and improving health and objectives for improving health. 2 vols.* Washington, DC: Government Printing Office.

HHS. 2008. *America's health literacy: Why we need accessible health information. An issue brief from the U.S. Department of Health and Human Services*. http://www.health.gov/communication/literacy/issuebrief/#intro (accessed July 20, 2009).

IOM (Institute of Medicine). 1988. *The future of public health*. Washington, DC: National Academy Press.

IOM. 1997. *Improving health in the community: A role for performance monitoring*. Washington, DC: National Academy Press.

IOM. 2003. *Speaking of health: Assessing health communication strategies for diverse populations.* Washington, DC: The National Academies Press.

IOM. 2004. *Health literacy: A prescription to end confusion.* Washington, DC: The National Academies Press.

Jacobson, K. 2008. *Strategies to improve communication between pharmacy staff and patients: A training program for pharmacy staff.* http://www.ahrq.gov/qual/pharmlit/pharmtrain. htm (accessed 2009).

Jiao, L., P. N. Mitrou, J. Reedy, B. I. Graubard, A. R. Hollenbeck, A. Schatzkin, and R. Stolzenberg-Solomon. 2009. A combined healthy lifestyle score and risk of pancreatic cancer in a large cohort study. *Archives of Internal Medicine* 169(8):764-770.

Kickbusch, I., and D. Maag. 2008. Health literacy. In *International encyclopedia of public health.* Vol. 3, edited by K. Heggenhougen and S. Quah. San Diego: Academic Press. Pp. 204-211.

McCormack, L., C. Bann, J. Uhrig, N. Berkman, and R. Rudd. 2009. Health insurance literacy of older adults. *Journal of Consumer Affairs* 43(2):223-248.

Moritsugu, K. 2006. In *Proceedings from the Surgeon General's workshop on improving health literacy.* http://www.surgeongeneral.gov/topics/healthliteracy/pdf/proceedings120607. pdf (accessed July 20, 2009).

Mozaffarian, D., A. Kamineni, M. Carnethon, L. Djousse, K. J. Mukamal, and D. Siscovick. 2009. Lifestyle risk factors and new-onset diabetes mellitus in older adults: The cardiovascular health study. *Archives of Internal Medicine* 169(8):798-807.

Mustard, J. F., and J. Frank. 1991. *The determinants of health.* Toronto: Canadian Institute of Advanced Research.

Nolan, T., and D. M. Berwick. 2006. All-or-none measurement raises the bar on performance. *JAMA: The Journal of the American Medical Association* 295(10):1168-1170.

Paasche-Orlow, M. K., D. Schillinger, S. M. Greene, and E. H. Wagner. 2006. How health care systems can begin to address the challenge of limited literacy. *Journal of General Internal Medicine* 21(8):884-887.

Pignone, M., D. A. DeWalt, S. Sheridan, N. Berkman, and K. N. Lohr. 2005. Interventions to improve health outcomes for patients with low literacy. A systematic review. *Journal of General Internal Medicine* 20(2):185-192.

Ratzan, S. C. 2009. In pursuit of health and happiness with global health diplomacy. *Journal of Health Communication: International Perspectives* 14(3):207-209.

Ratzan, S. C., and R. M. Parker. 2000. Introduction. In *National Library of Medicine current bibliographies in medicine: Health literacy,* edited by C. R. Selden, M. Zorn, S. C. Ratzan and R. M. Parker. Bethesda, MD: National Institutes of Health, U.S. Department of Health and Human Services.

Ratzan, S. C., G. L. Filerman, and J. W. LeSar. 2000. Attaining global health: Challenges and opportunities. *Population Bulletin* 55(1):1-48.

Rothman, R. L., R. Housam, H. Weiss, D. Davis, R. Gregory, T. Gebretsadik, A. Shintani, and T. A. Elasy. 2006. Patient understanding of food labels: The role of literacy and numeracy. *American journal of preventive medicine* 31(5):391-398.

Rudd, R. 2006. *Functional health literacy: Health information in everyday life.* In *Proceedings from the Surgeon General's workshop on improving health literacy.* http://www.surgeongeneral. gov/topics/healthliteracy/pdf/proceedings120607.pdf (accessed July 20, 2009).

Sanders, L. M., S. Federico, P. Klass, M. A. Abrams, and B. Dreyer. 2009. Literacy and child health: A systematic review. *Archives of Pediatric and Adolescent Medicine* 163(2):131-140.

Schillinger, D. 2006. *Literacy, chronic disease care, and public healthcare systems: A focus on communication. In proceedings from the surgeon general's workshop on improving health literacy.* http://www.surgeongeneral.gov/topics/healthliteracy/pdf/proceedings120607.pdf (accessed July 20, 2009).

Smith, E. 2008. Health journalists face translation challenge, Missouri journalism researchers find. *Missouri University News*, August 22, 2008.

Sudore, R. L., C. S. Landefeld, D. E. Barnes, K. Lindquist, B. A. Williams, R. Brody, and D. Schillinger. 2007. An advance directive redesigned to meet the literacy level of most adults: A randomized trial. *Patient Education and Counseling* 69(1-3):165-195.

Sudore, R. L., C. S. Landefeld, E. J. Perez-Stable, K. Bibbins-Domingo, B. A. Williams, and D. Schillinger. 2009. Unraveling the relationship between literacy, language proficiency, and patient-physician communication. *Patient Education and Counseling* 75(3):398-402.

Vernon, J. A., A. Trujillo, S. Rosenbaum, and B. DeBuono. 2007. *Low health literacy: Implications for national health policy.* http://www.gwumc.edu/sphhs/departments/healthpolicy/CHPR/downloads/LowHealthLiteracyReport10_4_07.pdf (accessed 2009).

Wallace, A. S., H. K. Seligman, T. C. Davis, D. Schillinger, C. L. Arnold, B. Bryant-Shilliday, J. K. Freburger, and D. A. DeWalt. 2009. Literacy-appropriate educational materials and brief counseling improve diabetes self-management. *Patient Education and Counseling* 75(3):328-333.

WHCA (World Health Communication Associates). 2009. *Health literacy, part 1 "the basics." WHCA action guide.* http://www.whcaonline.org/uploads/publications/WHCAhealthLiteracy-The%20Basics.pdf (accessed 2009).

Wolf, M. S., T. C. Davis, H. H. Tilson, P. F. Bass, and R. M. Parker. 2006. Misunderstanding of prescription drug warning labels among patients with low literacy. *American Journal of Health-System Pharmacy* 63(11):1048-1055.